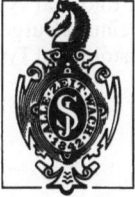

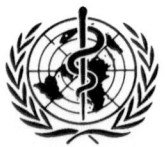 World Health Organization

---

The series *International Histological Classification of Tumours* consists of the following volumes. Each of these volumes – apart from volumes 1 and 2, which have already been revised – will appear in a revised edition within the next few years. Volumes of the current editions can be ordered through WHO, Distribution and Sales, Avenue Appia, CH-1211 Geneva 27.

1. Histological typing of lung tumours (1967, second edition 1981)
2. Histological typing of breast tumours (1968, second edition 1981)
3. Histological typing of soft tissue tumours (1969)
4. Histological typing of oral and oropharyngeal tumours (1971)
8. Cytology of the female genital tract (1973)
9. Histological typing of ovarian tumours (1973)
10. Histological typing of urinary bladder tumours (1973)
12. Histological typing of skin tumours (1974)
13. Histological typing of female genital tract tumours (1975)
14. Histological and cytological typing of neoplastic diseases
    of haematopoietic and lymphoid tissues (1976)
16. Histological typing of testis tumours (1977)
17. Cytology of non-gynaecological sites (1977)
20. Histological typing of tumours of the liver, biliary tract and pancreas (1978)
22. Histological typing of prostate tumours (1980)
23. Histological typing of endocrine tumours (1980)
24. Histological typing of tumours of the eye and its adnexa (1980)
25. Histological typing of kidney tumours (1981)

A coded compendium of the International Histological Classification of Tumours (1978).

The following volumes have already appeared in a revised edition with Springer-Verlag:

Histological Typing of Thyroid Tumours, 2nd edn. Hedinger/Williams/Sobin (1988)
Histological Typing of Intestinal Tumours, 2nd edn. Jass/Sobin (1989)
Histological Typing of Oesophageal and Gastric Tumours, 2nd edn.
Watanabe/ Jass/Sobin (1990)
Histological Typing of Tumours of the Gallbladder and Extrahepatic Bile Ducts,
2nd edn. Albores-Saavedra/Henson/Sobin (1990)
Histological Typing of Tumours of the Upper Respiratory Tract and Ear, 2nd edn.
Shanmugaratnam/Sobin (1991)
Histological Typing of Salivary Gland Tumours, 2nd edn. Seifert (1991)
Histological Typing of Odontogenic Tumours, 2nd edn. Kramer/Pindborg/Shear (1992)
Histological Typing of Tumours of the Central Nervous System, 2nd edn.
Kleihues/Burger/Scheithauer (1993)
Histological Typing of Bone Tumours, 2nd edn. Schajowicz (1993)

Histological Typing of Bone Tumours

F. Schajowicz

In Collaboration
with Pathologists in 9 Countries

Second Edition

With 166 Figures, Mostly in Colour

Springer-Verlag
Berlin Heidelberg New York
London Paris Tokyo
Hong Kong Barcelona
Budapest

F. Schajowicz †
Head, WHO Collaborating Centre
for the Histological Classification of Bone Tumours
Italian Hospital, Buenos Aires, Argentina
and Department of Orthopedic Surgery and Pathology
St. Louis University Medical Center, St. Louis, Missouri, USA

Series Editor
L. H. Sobin
Head, WHO Collaborating Centre
for the International Histological Classification of Tumours
Armed Forces Institute of Pathology, Washington, DC, USA

In this series, colour illustrations will be limited in number in order to maintain a reasonable sales price.

The printing of additional colour figures was made possible by financial support from Prof. F. J. Martinez-Tello, Madrid, Dr. T. Matsuno, Kita-Ku Sapporo, Prof. Dr. M. Salzer-Kuntschik, Vienna and the following Japanese companies: Daiichi Pharmacological Co., Howmedica, Mitsubishi Yuka Bio-clinical Laboratories Inc., Roussel Morishita KK, Taisho Pharmacological Co.

First edition published by WHO in 1972 as No. 6 in the International Histological Classification of Tumours series

ISBN-13:978-3-540-56460-7   e-ISBN-13:978-3-642-84902-2
DOI: 10.1007/978-3-642-84902-2

Library of Congress Cataloging-in-Publication Data
Schajowicz, Fritz. Histological typing of bone tumors / F. Schajowicz, in collaboration with pathologists in 9 countries. – 2nd ed. p. cm. – (International histological classification of tumors) Includes bibliographical references and index. ISBN-13:978-3-540-56460-7

1. Bones – Tumors – Histopathology. 2. Bones – Tumors – Classification. I. Title. II. Series: International historial classification of tumors (Unnumbered) [DNLM: 1. Bone Neoplasms – classification. 2. Bone Neoplasms – pathology. WE 258 S296h 1993] RC280.B6S318 1993 616.99'271'0014 – dc20 DNLM/DLC for Library of Congress 93-17622 CIP

Reproduction of the figures: Gustav Dreher GmbH, Stuttgart

21/3145-5 4 3 2 1 0 – Printed on acid-free paper

Histological Typing of Bone Tumours

F. Schajowicz

In Collaboration
with Pathologists in 9 Countries

Second Edition

With 166 Figures, Mostly in Colour

Springer-Verlag
Berlin Heidelberg New York
London Paris Tokyo
Hong Kong Barcelona
Budapest

F. Schajowicz †
Head, WHO Collaborating Centre
for the Histological Classification of Bone Tumours
Italian Hospital, Buenos Aires, Argentina
and Department of Orthopedic Surgery and Pathology
St. Louis University Medical Center, St. Louis, Missouri, USA

Series Editor
L. H. Sobin
Head, WHO Collaborating Centre
for the International Histological Classification of Tumours
Armed Forces Institute of Pathology, Washington, DC, USA

In this series, colour illustrations will be limited in number in order to maintain a reasonable sales price.

The printing of additional colour figures was made possible by financial support from Prof. F. J. Martinez-Tello, Madrid, Dr. T. Matsuno, Kita-Ku Sapporo, Prof. Dr. M. Salzer-Kuntschik, Vienna and the following Japanese companies: Daiichi Pharmacological Co., Howmedica, Mitsubishi Yuka Bio-clinical Laboratories Inc., Roussel Morishita KK, Taisho Pharmacological Co.

First edition published by WHO in 1972 as No. 6 in the International Histological Classification of Tumours series

ISBN-13:978-3-540-56460-7   e-ISBN-13:978-3-642-84902-2
DOI: 10.1007/978-3-642-84902-2

Library of Congress Cataloging-in-Publication Data
Schajowicz, Fritz. Histological typing of bone tumors / F. Schajowicz, in collaboration with pathologists in 9 countries. – 2nd ed. p. cm. – (International histological classification of tumors) Includes bibliographical references and index. ISBN-13:978-3-540-56460-7

1. Bones – Tumors – Histopathology. 2. Bones – Tumors – Classification. I. Title. II. Series: International historial classification of tumors (Unnumbered) [DNLM: 1. Bone Neoplasms – classification. 2. Bone Neoplasms – pathology. WE 258 S296h 1993] RC280.B6S318 1993 616.99'271'0014 – dc20 DNLM/DLC for Library of Congress 93-17622 CIP

© Springer-Verlag Berlin Heidelberg 1993

The use of general descriptive names, registered names, trademarks, etc. in this publication does not imply, even in the absence of a specific statement, that such names are exempt from the relevant protective laws and regulations and therefore free for general use.

Product liability: The publishers cannot guarantee the accuracy of any information about dosage and application contained in this book. In every individual case the user must check such information by consulting the relevant literature.

Reproduction of the figures: Gustav Dreher GmbH, Stuttgart

21/3145-5 4 3 2 1 0 – Printed on acid-free paper

Participants

Ackerman, L. V., M. D.
Department of Pathology, State University of New York at Stony
Brook, Stony Brook, New York, USA

Adler, C. P., M. D.
Pathologisches Institut der Universität Freiburg (Ludwig-Aschoff
Haus), Freiburg i. Br., FRG

Bertoni, F., M. D.
Anatomia Pathologia Malpighi, Bologna, Italy

Donato de Próspero, J., M. D.
Departamento Patológica Anatomía, Faculdade de Ciencias
Medicas de Santa Casa de São Paulo, Brazil

Martínez Tello, F. J., M. D.
Hospital "Primero de Octubre," Departamento de Anatomía
Patológica, Madrid, Spain

Mazabraud, A., M. D.
Pavillon Ollier, Hospital Cochin, Paris, France

Matsuno, T., M. D.
Department of Orthopaedics, Hokkaido University School
of Medicine, Kita-Ku, Sapporo, Japan

Povysil, C., M. D.
Second Department of Pathology, Charles University, Prague,
Czechoslovakia

Salzer-Kuntschik, M., M. D.
Institut für Pathologische Anatomie, Vienna, Austria

Schajowicz, F., M. D. †
Head, WHO Collaborating Centre for the Histological
Classification of Bone Tumours, Italian Hospital, Buenos Aires,
Argentina, *and* Department of Orthopedic Surgery
and Pathology, St. Louis University Medical Center, St. Louis,
Missouri, USA

Sissons, H. A., M. D.
Department of Pathology, Hospital for Joint Diseases, Orthopedic
Institute, New York, USA, *Present address:* Histopathology Unit,
Imperial Cancer Research Fund Laboratories,
Royal College of Surgeons of England, London, UK

Sobin, L. H., M. D.
Head, WHO Collaborating Centre for International Histological
Classification of Tumours, Armed Forces Institute of Pathology,
Washington, DC, USA

Unni, K. K., M. B., B. S.
Department of Surgical Pathology, Mayo Clinic, Rochester,
Minnesota, USA

General Preface to the Series

Among the prerequisites for comparative studies of cancer are international agreement on histological criteria for the definition and classification of cancer types and a standardized nomenclature. An internationally agreed classification of tumours, acceptable alike to physicians, surgeons, radiologists, pathologists and statisticians, would enable cancer workers in all parts of the world to compare their findings and would facilitate collaboration among them.

In a report published in 1952,[1] a subcommittee of the World Health Organization (WHO) Expert Committee on Health Statistics discussed the general principles that should govern the statistical classification of tumours and agreed that, to ensure the necessary flexibility and ease of coding, three separate classifications were needed according to (1) anatomical site, (2) histological type, and (3) degree of malignancy. A classification according to anatomical site is available in the International Classification of Diseases.[2]

In 1956, the WHO Executive Board passed a resolution[3] requesting the Director-General to explore the possibility that WHO might organize centres in various parts of the world and arrange for the collection of human tissues and their histological classification. The main purpose of such centres would be to develop histological definitions of cancer types and to facilitate the wide adoption of a uniform nomenclature. The resolution was endorsed by the Tenth World Health Assembly in May 1957.[4]

---

[1] WHO (1952) WHO Technical Report Series. No. 53, 1952, p 45
[2] WHO (1977) Manual of the international statistical classification of diseases, injuries, and causes of death, 1975 version. Geneva
[3] WHO (1956) WHO Official Records. No. 68, p 14 (resolution EB 17.R40)
[4] WHO (1957) WHO Official Records. No. 79, p 467 (resolution WHA 10.18)

Since 1958, WHO has established a number of centres concerned with this subject. The result of this endeavour has been the International Histological Classification of Tumours, a multivolumed series whose first edition was published between 1967 and 1981. The present revised second edition aims to update the classification, reflecting progress in diagnosis and the relevance of tumour types to clinical and epidemiological features.

Preface to Histological Typing of Bone Tumours, Second Edition

The first edition of *Histological Typing of Bone Tumours*[1] was the result of a collaborative effort organized by WHO and carried out by the International Reference/Collaborating Centre for the Histological Classification of Bone Tumours at the Osteo-Articular Pathology Centre, Italian Hospital, Buenos Aires, Argentina. The Centre was established in 1963, and the classification was published in 1972.

In order to keep the classification up to date, the Centre circulated a set of revision proposals to the participants listed on pages V and VI. Their reponses provided the basis for a new draft. After further communications among the participants, the present classification, definitions and explanatory notes were recommended for publication.

Professor Schajowicz, Head of the WHO Centre, died suddenly during the final stages of preparation of the publication. His former pupil and colleague, Dr. H. Gallardo, Spanish Hospital, Buenos Aires, Argentina, helped to complete the selection of illustrations. Dr. K. Shanmugaratnam, Singapore, Head of the WHO Centre for Upper Respiratory Tract Tumours, and Dr. Sharon Weiss, Ann Arbor, Head of the WHO Centre for Soft Tissue Tumours, reviewed the final draft of the manuscript and provided valuable comments.

The histological classification of bone tumours, which appears on pages 3–6, contains the morphology code numbers of the International Classification of Diseases for Oncology (ICD-O)[2] and the Systematized Nomenclature of Medicine (SNOMED).[3]

---

[1] Schajowicz F, Ackerman VL, Sissons HA, Sobin LH, Torloni H (1972) Histological Typing of Bone Tumours. Geneva, World Health Organization (International Histological Classification of Tumours, No. 6)
[2] World Health Organization (1990) International Classification of Diseases for Oncology. Geneva
[3] College of American Pathologists (1982) Systematized Nomenclature of Medicine. Chicago

It will, of course, be appreciated that the classification reflects the present state of knowledge, and modifications are almost certain to be needed as experience accumulates. Although the present classification has been adopted by the members of the group, it necessarily represents a view from which some pathologists may wish to dissent. It is nevertheless hoped that, in the interests of international cooperation, all pathologists will use the classification as put forward. Criticism and suggestions for its improvement will be welcomed; these should be sent to the World Health Organization, Geneva, Switzerland.

The publications in the series *International Histological Classification of Tumours* are not intended to serve as textbooks but rather to promote the adoption of a uniform terminology that will facilitate communication among cancer workers. For this reason the literature references have intentionally been omitted and readers should refer to standard works for bibliographies.

Contents

Introduction

During the two decades since the publication of the first edition of *Histological Typing of Bone Tumours,* new methods of diagnosis, especially radiological imaging techniques (computed tomography and magnetic resonance imaging), associated with advances in the new cytomorphological methods including immunohistochemistry, DNA ploidy analysis, cytogenetic chromosomal investigation, etc., have greatly improved our diagnostic tools and treatment results. These advances are reflected by the publication of new editions of various important textbooks in recent years. In these publications classification criteria differed.

In contrast, the WHO classification has been relatively unaltered, and has introduced a limited number of new entities and subdivided others because of distinct histological features and biological behaviour.

In general the framework and the concept of the original classification, as it has been widely accepted, remains essentially unchanged. The classification is based on the line of histological differentiation, in many instances reflecting the type of intercellular matrix material produced. This approach is justified because it avoids theoretical histogenetic controversies.

The classification includes benign and malignant neoplasms primary in bone, together with certain "tumor-like" lesions that were introduced because of their importance in differential diagnosis and because of uncertainty regarding their neoplastic nature. It is true that the number of lesions in this category could be widened to include an endless number of lesions simulating bone tumours based on clinical-radiographic findings. Some of these lesions are relatively common (Paget disease, fracture callus, osteomyelitis, osteonecrosis) and others are extremely rare (melorheostosis, congenital or acquired osseous dysplasia, massive osteolysis, etc.). In order to simplify the classification, only a reduced group of relatively frequent lesions located within bone or on its surface which may present problems of differential diagnosis are included. Metastatic and soft tissue tumours have been excluded.

The diagnosis of a bone lesion should be established by a combination of clinical, radiological and pathological studies. Therefore, the typical radiographic images are included with the pathological findings.

Most bone tumours can be diagnosed by routine haematoxylin-eosin stains, but in some cases immunohistochemical studies are needed.

Although this revised classification reflects the present state of knowledge, modifications undoubtedly will be needed in the future. Hopefully the adoption of a uniform terminology will continue to facilitate communication among oncologists.

Histological Classification of Bone Tumours

1   Bone-forming tumours

1.1   *Benign*
1.1.1   Osteoma................................. 9180/0[a]
1.1.2   Osteoid osteoma and osteoblastoma
1.1.2.1   Osteoid osteoma.......................... 9191/0
1.1.2.2   Osteoblastoma 9200/0

1.2   *Intermediate*
1.2.1   Aggressive (malignant) osteoblastoma 9200/1

1.3   *Malignant*
1.3.1   Osteosarcoma 9180/3
1.3.1.1   Central (medullary) osteosarcoma 9180/3
1.3.1.1.1 Conventional central osteosarcoma 9180/3
1.3.1.1.2 Telangiectatic osteosarcoma 9183/3
1.3.1.1.3 Intraosseous well-differentiated (low-grade)
          osteosarcoma............................. 9180/31
1.3.1.1.4 Round-cell osteosarcoma 9185/3
1.3.1.2   Surface osteosarcoma 9190/3
1.3.1.2.1 Parosteal (juxtacortical) osteosarcoma 9190/31
1.3.1.2.2 Periosteal osteosarcoma 9190/32
1.3.1.2.3 High-grade surface osteosarcoma 9190/33

2   Cartilage-forming tumours

2.1   *Benign*
2.1.1   Chondroma 9220/0
2.1.1.1   Enchondroma 9220/0
2.1.1.2   Periosteal (juxtacortical) chondroma.......... 9221/0

---

[a] Morphology code of the International Classification of Diseases for Oncology (ICD-O) and the Systematized Nomenclature of Medicine (SNOMED).

Definitions and Explanatory Notes

1 Bone-Forming Tumours

1.1 Benign

1.1.1 Osteoma (Figs. 1–3)

A benign, slowly growing lesion consisting of well-differentiated mature bone, with a predominantly lamellar structure.

These lesions are regarded by some as hamartomas rather than true neoplasms. Three different types of osteoma are distinguished: conventional osteoma ("ivory exostosis"), parosteal (juxtacortical) osteoma, and medullary osteoma (bone island or enostoma).

Conventional osteoma is almost entirely restricted to bones of intramembranous (direct) bone formation, that is, the external table of the skull and the paranasal sinuses, where it appears as a dense ivory-like bony mass. The location at the inner table and maxillary bones is less frequent and only rarely is the external surface of a long or flat bone involved (parosteal or juxtacortical osteoma).

Lesions with similar histological features found in the medullary cavity of other bones are called "medullary osteomas" (or "enostomas" or "bone islands"). They generally present as radiological findings without clinical relevance or growth potential and are considered as hamartomas.

1.1.2 Osteoid Osteoma and Osteoblastoma

Osteoid osteoma and osteoblastoma are closely related entities of osteoblastic type and appear under a common heading. At one time, the term "giant osteoid osteoma" was used (but later abandoned) for benign osteoblastoma to convey the relationship between the lesions.

Although there are no specific histological criteria to distinguish between them, the two terms are retained because of their wide acceptance based on differences in the size, site, radiological appearance, clinical presentation and surrounding bony reaction. It is possible that these differences are related to the respective sites of the two lesions: cortical for osteoid osteoma and medullary for osteoblastoma.

Considering both lesions as closely related tumours of osteoblastoma derivation, the terms "circumscribed" or "cortical" osteoblastoma for conventional osteoid osteoma, and "genuine" or "spongious" osteoblastoma for osteoblastoma have been proposed.

1.1.2.1 Osteoid Osteoma (Figs. 4–8)

A benign osteoblastic lesion characterized by its small size (usually less than 1 cm), a clearly demarcated outline, and usually the presence of a surrounding zone of reactive bone formation. Histologically, it consists of immature bone and osteoid within a cellular, highly vascularized stroma.

An arbitrary criterion generally used to determine whether a lesion is diagnosed as osteoid osteoma or osteoblastoma is the size of the nidus: lesions less than 1 or 2 cm in diameter are classified as osteoid osteoma; those larger are osteoblastoma. Others have used a dividing line of 1.5 cm for lesions indistinguishable by all other criteria.

Osteoid osteoma typically occurs in the shaft of long bones, particularly the tibia and femur, the femoral neck and intertrochanteric region accounting for most of them. Unlike osteoblastoma, osteoid osteoma is infrequent in the spine. The majority of osteoid osteomas occur during the second decade of life with a predilection for males (3:1). Pain is the most common clinical manifestation, often worse in the evening and relieved by salicylates. Osteoid osteoma may have an intrarticular location and present as synovitis of the involved joint. Multiple loci or a subperiosteal location are extremely rare.

Radioisotope imaging and computed tomography are very useful in both anatomical localization and diagnosis.

1.1.2.2 Osteoblastoma (Figs. 9–11)

A benign or locally aggressive tumour with a histological structure similar to that of osteoid osteoma, but characterized by its larger size (usually more than 1.5 cm) and typically by the absence of a surrounding zone of conspicuous reactive bone formation.

Osteoblastomas are less frequent than osteoid osteomas. They most frequently occur in the vertebrae and flat bones, and in the bones of the hand or foot; they do not, as a rule, produce the intense pain commonly associated with osteoid osteoma. They occur more frequently in males, and during the first three decades of life.

There is a diversity in the natural history, i. e. malignant potential, of osteoblastoma; conventional osteoblastoma should be considered an unpredictable lesion. The term "benign" therefore should not be used.

1.2 Intermediate

1.2.1 Aggressive (Malignant) Osteoblastoma (Figs. 12–14)

An osteoblastoma with abundant and large hypertrophic osteoblasts, often having plump or bizarre hyperchromatic nuclei and alternating fields of giant cells of osteoclastic type. These lesions contain "blue spiculated bone" produced by typical osteoblasts.

Conventional osteoblastomas have a significant recurrence rate of approximately 15 %, especially after intralesional excision (curettage). Although very rare, cases have been reported of malignant transformation to typical osteosarcoma.

The histological distinction from osteosarcoma may be difficult. However, in the type of osteoblastoma designated "malignant osteoblastoma" (Schajowicz and Lemos), the areas of necrosis, atypical mitosis and malignant cartilage so evident in osteosarcoma are lacking. Lesions with similar distinctive histological features have been designated "aggressive osteoblastoma" (Dorfman).

In spite of their more aggressive clinical course and frequent recurrence, none of the lesions reported as "malignant" or "aggressive" osteoblastoma have metastasized. Therefore, as the lesions appear to have no metastatic potential, the name "aggressive osteoblastoma" seems more appropriate. The term "osteosarcoma in situ" has recently been suggested. Wide excision, preferably en bloc, is the indicated treatment.

1.3 Malignant

1.3.1 Osteosarcoma (Figs. 15–44)

A malignant tumour characterized by the direct formation of bone or osteoid by the tumour cells.

The term "osteosarcoma" is now increasingly being used by most centres, replacing the older term "osteogenic sarcoma". Osteosarcoma is the most common primary malignant tumour of bone apart from myeloma. It covers a wide spectrum of lesions with distinct clinical and pathological features, associated with different biological behaviours. Two fundamental groups can be clearly separated, the central (medullary) and the surface (peripheral) osteosarcomas. Intracortical osteosarcomas are extremely rare and only isolated cases have been reported.

1.3.1.1 Central (Medullary) Osteosarcoma (Figs. 15–21)

Besides the more common conventional or classic osteosarcoma, several variants of central osteosarcoma have been described: the telangiectatic osteosarcoma, the well-differentiated (low-grade) osteosarcoma, and the small-cell osteosarcoma simulating Ewing sarcoma. With the exception of the well-differentiated osteosarcoma, all are highly malignant.

1.3.1.1.1 Conventional Central Osteosarcoma

An osteosarcoma that arises centrally and after destroying the cortex invades the surrounding tissues, but generally respects the adjacent growth cartilage.

Grossly and radiographically, an almost purely sclerosing and an osteolytic variety may be distinguished; however, a mixture of these features is more common.

Osteosarcomas show considerable variation in gross and histological pattern, differing greatly in the amount of tumour bone or osteoid present, in the pleomorphism of the tumour tissue and in the number of atypical mitoses and extent of necrosis. In addition to bone and osteoid, the tumour cells may produce cartilage, fibrous tissue or myxoid tissue; many areas of tumour tissue may have an undifferentiated spindle-celled structure without any specific type of intercellular material. Subdivision of osteosarcomas on the basis of a predominantly osteoblastic, chondroblastic, fibroblastic or fibrohistiocytic structure can be useful for recognition but does not seem to be of importance as far as prognosis and treatment are concerned.

Most tumours occur in patients between the ages of 10 and 20 years; they are relatively infrequent below the age of 10 years and exceptional under 5 years and over 40 years of age. Many of the tumours developing after middle age are associated with Paget disease of bone (Figs. 22–24) or, more rarely, following irradiation or secondary to fibrous dysplasia. Males are more frequently affected than females. The metaphysis of the long bones, particularly the lower end of the femur, the upper end of the tibia and the upper end of the humerus (that is, areas near the most actively growing epiphysis) are the sites of predilection.

1.3.1.1.2 Telangiectatic Osteosarcoma (Figs. 25–28)
An osteosarcoma characterized by numerous large spaces filled with blood and separated by fibrous septa.

There are areas of conspicuous cellular anaplasia frequently associated with giant cells of the osteoclast type or with atypical multinucleated giant cells. Tumour osteoid or bone is often scarce and may be difficult to find. Therefore, this lesion is often mistaken for an aneurysmal bone cyst or a malignant giant cell tumour. Radiologically, telangiectatic osteosarcoma appears as a moth-eaten or permeative radiolucent lesion, most commonly located in the metadiaphyseal region. On gross examination the tumour is a haemorrhagic multiloculated mass. Following these criteria this neoplasm is relatively rare (approximately 1 % of all osteosarcomas). The particularly poor prognosis associated with this tumour in earlier times has improved due to new pre- and postoperative chemotherapeutic methods.

1.3.1.1.3 Intraosseous Well-Differentiated (Low-Grade) Osteosarcoma (Figs. 29–31)
An osteosarcoma composed mainly of fibrous and osseous tissue with little cellular atypia or mitotic activity.

This has been identified in recent years as a distinct entity with a better prognosis than the conventional central osteosarcoma. It has many histological similarities to parosteal (juxtacortical) osteosarcoma and shares its biological behaviour. In some cases the histological features may simulate fibrous dysplasia or aggressive osteoblastoma. This variant of osteosarcoma is rare and comprises approximately 1 % of all osteosarcomas.

1.3.1.1.4 Round-Cell Osteosarcoma (Figs. 32–34)

An osteosarcoma with the histological features of both Ewing sarcoma and osteosarcoma.

This rare variant (about 1 % of osteosarcomas) has been labelled "small-cell or round-cell osteosarcoma simulating Ewing sarcoma". Recognition of this rare entity is important because of possible differences in response to treatment.

1.3.1.2 Surface Osteosarcoma (Figs. 35–44)

An osteosarcoma that arises from the surface of the bone.

Surface osteosarcomas occur mostly in long bones and are far less common than those arising within bone. They can be subdivided into three categories: parosteal (juxtacortical), periosteal and high-grade surface osteosarcoma. This division is justified because of differences in histological features, biological behaviour and prognosis. Parosteal osteosarcoma is associated with the best prognosis; high-grade surface osteosarcoma has a poor prognosis, almost identical to that of conventional central osteosarcoma. The prognosis of periosteal osteosarcoma is intermediate.

1.3.1.2.1 Parosteal (Juxtacortical) Osteosarcoma (Figs. 35–38)

A distinct type of osteosarcoma, characterized by an origin on the external surface of a bone and a high degree of structural differentiation.

These tumours grow relatively slowly and have a better prognosis than the ordinary type of osteosarcoma. Histologically, the tumour consists of a mass of bone trabeculae, often mature and lamellar. The trabeculae are separated by fibrous tissue composed of spindle cells that are minimally pleomorphic and have few mitoses. Occasionally, at the periphery of the tumour, small areas of cartilage show the histological pattern of low-grade chondrosarcoma. The distinction from myositis ossificans may be difficult, particularly with a parosteal osteosarcoma at an early stage of development.

The term "parosteal osteosarcoma" is at present preferred to the older term "juxtacortical osteosarcoma" used by Jaffe. This is to avoid confusion, since some authorities have grouped all surface osteosarcomas under the single title of "juxtacortical osteosarcoma".

Parosteal osteosarcoma usually spares the medullary cavity unless the lesion is of long duration or has had surgical treatment. These tumours usually occur in young adults and involve the shafts of long bones, most commonly the lower and posterior part of the femur and the upper part of the humerus. They are circumscribed and sometimes lobulated lesions, adherent to or surrounding the cortex of the bone. They are relatively infrequent tumours (10 % of all osteosarcomas).

According to the above definition, highly malignant surface tumours, previously regarded as grade III parosteal osteosarcomas, should be classified as high-grade surface osteosarcomas. In some tumours, especially after a recurrence, areas of high-grade malignancy may be found in an otherwise well-differentiated lesion: these lesions have been called "dedifferentiated" parosteal osteosarcomas.

1.3.1.2.2 Periosteal Osteosarcoma (Figs. 39–41)

A surface osteosarcoma that contains predominantly low- or medium-grade malignant cartilage, often undergoing calcification or enchondral ossification. In focal areas, the tumour produces fine lace-like osteoid.

Although long recognized, periosteal osteosarcoma has been more clearly defined in the last decade. It occurs most often in adolescents and has a predilection for the diaphyses of the femur and tibia. There is only occasional involvement of the underlying cortex, and penetration of the medullary cavity is rare. In at least some patients the tumour resembles periosteal chondrosarcoma, an entity with similar clinical and radiographic features. Areas that have been interpreted as lace-like osteoid or tumour bone may actually be strands of cartilage or areas of enchondral ossification.

1.3.1.2.3 High-Grade Surface Osteosarcoma (Figs. 42–44)

A surface osteosarcoma with highly malignant histological features.

This lesion occurs most frequently in adolescents and is predominantly located in the diaphyses of long bones, mostly in the femur or humerus. The radiographic features may be similar to those of periosteal osteosarcoma. The prognosis is almost as bad as that of a conventional central osteosarcoma.

2 Cartilage-Forming Tumours

2.1 Benign

2.1.1 Chondroma (Figs. 45–47)

A benign tumour characterized by the formation of mature cartilage, but lacking the histological characteristics of chondrosarcoma (high cellularity, pleomorphism and presence of large cells with double nuclei or mitoses).

Benign cartilage tumours are relatively common lesions. Typically, they involve the short tubular bones of the hands and feet, and less commonly the ribs or the major long bones. They are usually situated centrally *(enchondroma);* periosteal (juxtacortical) chondromas are less frequent. The lesions may be solitary or part of the condition multiple enchondromatosis, in which several or many bones are affected. Cases of multiple enchondromatosis with a predominantly unilateral distribution are generally referred to as "Ollier disease" or "dyschondroplasia". When multiple enchondromas are accompanied by multiple hemangiomas of soft tissues, the term "Maffucci syndrome" is used.

Grossly, chondromas have a lobulated cartilaginous appearance. They often show necrosis and calcification, with or without enchondral ossification, and this may be evident radiologically. Myxoid change is common.

The histological distinction between chondroma and chondrosarcoma is sometimes difficult, particularly when only a limited sample of tissue is available. Lack of high cellularity, pleomorphism and plump cells with large or double nuclei favour a benign lesion. The site of the tumour and the radiological and clinical features are often helpful in making the distinction between benign and malignant cartilage tumours. Radiologically, enchondroma is radiolucent, often well-defined round or ovoid, expanding and slightly thinning the cortex. The lesion is usually located in the metaphysis, extending toward the diaphysis. Varying degrees of mottled calcification are common. There are often discrepancies between biological behaviour and histological appearance, depending on the clinical symptoms and the anatomical site of the lesion. Thus, solitary tumours of the tubular bones of the hands and feet and some periosteal tumours, although showing cytological features of low-grade malignancy, behave in a benign fashion.

Heavily calcified cartilaginous lesions that sometimes occur in the metaphyses of long bones, often without symptoms, have been referred to as "calcifying and ossifying chondromas". They are probably chondromatous hamartomas and not true neoplasms.

Malignant change is rare in a solitary enchondroma, particularly in the hands or feet, but occurs more frequently (in approximately 30 % of cases) in cases of multiple enchondromatosis, particularly in cases of Ollier or Maffucci syndrome.

2.1.2 Osteochondroma (Osteocartilaginous Exostosis)
(Figs. 48–51)

A cartilage-capped bony projection on the external surface of a bone.

This is a frequent type of bone lesion. It may be solitary or part of the generalized condition multiple hereditary exostoses ("diaphyseal aclasis" or "hereditary deforming chondrodysplasia"). Osteochondromas are commonly located in the metaphyseal regions of long bones, particularly the lower femur, upper tibia and upper humerus, but are also found in other bones such as the scapula or ilium. Solitary lesions may have either a broad or a narrow base (i. e. they may be either sessile or pedunculated), while multiple lesions can involve the whole metaphysis of a bone. Osteochondromas occur most frequently in children; their growth usually ceases at the time of skeletal maturation. They are probably disorders of growth rather than true neoplasms.

Malignant change is rare in solitary osteochondromas, but occurs more frequently (approximately 5 %) in cases of multiple hereditary osteochondromas.

2.1.3 Chondroblastoma (Epiphyseal Chondroblastoma)
(Figs. 52–55)

An uncommon benign tumour, characterized by highly cellular and relatively immature, rounded or polygonal, chondroblast-like cells with distinct outlines, together with multinucleated osteoclast-like giant cells arranged singly or in groups. On the whole, there is little intercellular material, but small amounts of cartilaginous intercellular matrix with areas of focal calcification are typical.

The lesions are almost invariably situated in the epiphyses of long bones adjacent to the epiphyseal cartilage plate; they sometimes extend into the adjacent metaphysis. The upper tibia, femur and upper humerus are common sites. The tumours usually occur in patients under 20 years of age. Codman in 1931 was the first to give a detailed account of this tumour, which he regarded as an "epiphyseal chondromatous giant cell tumor". In 1942, Jaffe and Lichtenstein suggested that the lesion was a specific type of tumour, distinct from giant cell tumour, and proposed the name "benign chondroblastoma". The distinction between chondroblastoma and chondromyxoid fibroma is not always clear, inasmuch as cases with some of the histological features of both have been reported. Cases with some of the histological features of aneurysmal bone cyst have been referred to as "cystic chondroblastoma".

A few cases of chondroblastoma may pursue a more aggressive course and recur locally with invasion of joint spaces and adjacent bone and/or soft tissue, but many of these developments are to be attributed to incorrect initial treatment. The existence of a "primary malignant chondroblastoma" is still questionable. The exceptional cases of malignant evolution which have been reported may be divided into the following categories: (1) Chondroblastoma with sarcomatous transformation, with or without prior radiation therapy ("secondary" malignant tumours). (2) Chondroblastoma exhibiting benign-appearing lung metastases. These metastases usually develop subsequent to surgery. They usually behave in a relatively benign fashion, with the exception of the one reported by Kyriakos et al.,[1] which pursued a malignant course. Unfortunately there are as yet no histological parameters that permit determination of which metastases will cease their growth or which will progress and kill the host. (3) Chondroblastoma-like chondrosarcoma, i.e. a chondrosarcoma resembling a chondroblastoma.

2.1.4 Chondromyxoid Fibroma (Figs. 56–59)

A benign tumour characterized by lobulated areas of spindle-shaped or stellate cells with abundant myxoid or chondroid intercellular material, separated by zones of more cellular tissue rich in spindle-shaped or rounded cells with a varying number of multinucleated giant cells of different sizes. Large pleomorphic cells may be present and can result in confusion with chondrosarcoma. However, atypical mitoses are lacking.

---

[1] Kyriakos M, Land VJ, Penning L et al. (1985) Metastatic chondroblastoma: report of a fatal case with a review of the literature on atypical, aggressive, and malignant chondroblastoma. Cancer 55: 1770–1789

These lesions are usually situated in the metaphyseal region of a long bone, particularly the upper tibia, and produce an expansion of part of the cortex. Lesions of the tarsal and metatarsal bones are not infrequent. The patients are adolescents or young adults, males and females being affected in equal numbers. Radiologically, the lesions appear as eccentric, sharply outlined, radiolucent areas that often cause expansion of the bone. They have a thin sclerotic inner border. Prior to the description of chondromyxoid fibroma these cases were often diagnosed as myxomas or chondromyxomas. Except in the jaws, true myxomas of bone very rarely, if ever, occur.

As noted, occasional tumours show a combination of the histological features of chondromyxoid fibroma and chondroblastoma.

The lesions may recur after curettage, but malignant change is extremely rare.

2.2 Malignant

2.2.1 Chondrosarcoma (Figs. 60–69)

A malignant tumour characterized by the formation of cartilage, but not of bone, by the tumour cells. It is distinguished from chondroma by its higher cellularity, greater pleomorphism and appreciable numbers of plump cells with large or double nuclei. Mitotic cells are infrequent.

Chondrosarcomas show wide variation in their clinical and histological features and behaviour, and several different variants besides the conventional central chondrosarcoma may be observed.

Chondrosarcomas are relatively common. They usually occur in patients between 30 and 60 years of age, and are rare in individuals under 20 years. In contrast to benign cartilaginous tumours, the majority of which occur toward the periphery of the limb, chondrosarcomas are found mainly in the pelvis, femur, ribs, shoulder girdle and humerus.

Chondrosarcomas usually originate in the central tissue of a bone (however, see Sect. 2.2.2 on juxtacortical chondrosarcoma). Some arise *de novo;* others, sometimes referred to as secondary chondrosarcomas, have their origin in a pre-existing benign cartilage tumour, most frequently in multiple hereditary exostoses (peripheral or exostotic chondrosarcoma) or multiple enchondromatosis (Ollier disease) Figs. 68, 69).

The histological distinction between benign and malignant cartilage tumours is sometimes difficult. The following criteria are helpful in diagnosing chondrosarcoma: plump and multinucleated cartilage cells, the permeation of the tumour through host cancellous bone, replacing marrow and trapping or encasing the host bone's lamellar trabeculae on all sides and endosteal scalloping and/or focal cortical destruction, often associated with cortical thickening. Chondrosarcomas are quite variable in their histological structure and behaviour, and an attempt should always be made to distinguish between slowly growing and relatively benign, well-differentiated lesions on one hand, and rapidly growing, more malignant, poorly differentiated tumours on the other.

Tumours with more or less conspicuous myxoid areas should not be confused with the so-called myxoid chondrosarcoma, an entity with distinctive histological and ultrastructural features not infrequently found primarily in the deep soft tissues of the extremities, but extremely rare within bone. They have also been referred to as "chordoid sarcoma".

The tissue of a chondrosarcoma frequently shows areas of calcification and enchondral ossification, but bone formation by the tumour cells is seen only in osteosarcoma.

2.2.2 Juxtacortical (Periosteal) Chondrosarcoma (Figs. 70–72)

A malignant cartilage-forming tumour arising from the external surface of a bone, possibly of periosteal origin, usually characterized by well-differentiated lobulated cartilage with extensive areas of spotty calcification and enchondral ossification; however, tumour osteoid or bone is absent.

Lesions of this type are rare, and possibly represent a cartilage counterpart of periosteal osteosarcoma. The lesion involves the shaft of a long bone, most often the femur, and occurs in adolescents, with a predominance in males. Characteristically, the tumour is small and adjacent to the cortex; sometimes it shows areas of spotty calcification, radiating bone spicules and often a typical Codman triangle. These tumours have a better prognosis than the similar central type of chondrosarcoma. A juxtacortical (periosteal) chondrosarcoma must be distinguished from a chondrosarcoma arising as a result of malignant change in the cartilage of an osteochondroma (peripheral or exostotic chondrosarcoma), a change more commonly associated with multiple hereditary osteochondromas.

2.2.3 Mesenchymal Chondrosarcoma (Figs. 73–75)

A malignant tumour, characterized by the presence of scattered areas of more or less differentiated cartilage together with highly vascular spindle-cell or round-cell "mesenchymal" tissue, often with a haemangiopericytomatous pattern.

These tumours are relatively rare, but have characteristic histological features which justify their separation as a distinctive malignant cartilage tumour. They are generally highly malignant; nearly one-third originate in juxtaosseous soft tissue; multifocal lesions have rarely been reported.

2.2.4 Dedifferentiated Chondrosarcoma (Figs. 76–78)

A highly anaplastic sarcoma juxtaposed to a borderline or low-grade malignant cartilage tumour. There is typically an abrupt transition between the components.

"Dedifferentiation" of a histologically low grade and clinically indolent cartilage tumour occurs in approximately 10 % of all chondrosarcomas. Although there is a question over the accuracy of the concept of dedifferentiation in the pathogenesis of this tumour, the term "dedifferentiated chondrosarcoma" continues to be used as a distinct, well-defined entity because it remains useful to indicate the tumour's more aggressive and malignant behaviour and poor prognosis. The tumour involves most frequently the long bones, particularly the femur, humerus, and pelvis; almost all are associated with a central chondrosarcoma. There is a wide range of age from 20 to 80 years.

2.2.5 Clear-Cell Chondrosarcoma (Figs. 79–81)

A tumour of low-grade malignancy characterized by rounded cells with conspicuous clear or vacuolated cytoplasm and by a cartilaginous or chondroid matrix in at least some areas. Scattered osteoclast-type giant cells, occasional bone trabeculae and aneurysmal bone cyst-like areas may be present.

Clear-cell chondrosarcoma is considered by some as a rare variety of chondrosarcoma, and by others as an atypical, more aggressive chondroblastoma or its malignant counterpart. It usually affects adults, most commonly involving the proximal part of the femur, humerus or tibia. These are sites similar to those of chondroblastoma, which often shows similar radiographic features. Clear-cell chondrosarcomas often recur after simple curettage but rarely metastasize; therefore a more aggressive treatment (resection) than that used for chondroblastoma has been advocated.

2.2.6 Malignant Chondroblastoma (Figs. 82–84)

The existence of this entity is questionable. For discussion see Sect. 2.1.3, chondroblastoma.

3 Giant-Cell Tumour (Osteoclastoma) (Figs. 85–95)

An aggressive tumour, characterized by richly vascularized tissue consisting of rather plump spindle-shaped or ovoid cells and by the presence of numerous giant cells of osteoclast type, which are uniformly distributed throughout the tumour tissue. There is relatively little collagen. Areas of haemorrhage and of regressive changes, such as necrosis, fibrosis and fibrohistiocytic reaction, are frequently present, especially in larger or longstanding tumours.

Most giant-cell tumours occur in patients between 20 and 40 years of age. They are rarely seen in patients below the age of 15 years and are extremely rare under the age of 10 years; this helps to distinguish them from certain benign lesions that were previously regarded as giant-cell tumours or variants (chondroblastoma, chondromyxoid fibroma, aneurysmal bone cyst, metaphyseal fibrous defect), but are now regarded as separate entities. Giant-cell tumours typically involve the ends of the long bones, common sites being the lower end of the femur, the upper end of the tibia and the lower end of the radius. The tumours are osteolytic. They originate towards the medial or lateral aspects of the ends of the bones, close to the articular cartilage; later the tumour occupies and even expands the entire end of the bone and the adjacent metaphysis. Men and women are affected with about equal frequency.

Giant-cell tumours can no longer be considered innocent growths. They present with few exceptions as aggressive, potentially malignant lesions that recur in about 20%–50% of patients after incisional excision (curettage), undergo sarcomatous transformation in about 5%–10% of patients, and even produce in rare instances pulmonary metastases without histological evidence of malignant changes. Synonyms have been "low-grade neoplastic giant cell tumour" or "semimalignant giant-cell tumour".

Cases of apparently metaphyseal origin in adolescent patients with an immature skeleton occur rarely. There are also some exceptional cases with a diaphyseal location.

In the past, attempts were made to histologically "grade" the tumours into benign, aggressive and malignant variants. These criteria have not proved to be satisfactory, however, and there is today no agreement on specific histological features that dependably indicate the likelihood of malignant behaviour. In this sense, all giant-cell tumours are potentially malignant. At present it is not possible to predict clinical behaviour on the basis of histological structure, and thus distinguish between "benign" and "malignant" varieties. The radiographic features dividing giant-cell tumours into three categories (grade I, quiescent; grade II, active; and grade III, aggressive) seem to be more important than histology for prognosis and treatment. Many cases of the quiescent radiological type, which generally have a more favourable prognosis, show a predominantly fibroxanthomatous histological pattern, and rarely if ever recur after excision.

So-called primary malignant giant-cell tumours seem to be extremely rare, and no clear histological criteria for their diagnosis have been established. The apparent incidence varies widely in different institutions. In most cases malignant change has occurred subsequent to the presence of a histologically verified benign tumour ("secondary" malignant giant cell tumour). The therapy has included irradiation in almost every instance; only in exceptional cases has the malignant tumour, usually a fibrosarcoma or osteosarcoma, developed after curettage only. Most other cases reported as "primary malignant giant-cell tumour", in which zones of typical benign giant-cell tumour tissue are present in association with some other type of clearly malignant neoplasm, are more likely other types of sarcoma that happen to be richly endowed with multinucleated giant cells of the osteoclastic type. The majority of these neoplasms appear to be telangiectatic or giant-cell-rich osteosarcomas, fibrosarcomas or malignant fibrous histiocytomas. Primary diffusely malignant giant-cell tumour with a roentgenogram consistent with the diagnosis of typical giant-cell tumour is extremely unusual.

Multicentric bone involvement by giant-cell tumours is unusual and may appear simultaneously or metachronously. It is necessary to exclude hyperparathyroidism.

The histogenesis of giant-cell tumour is still unclear. The giant cells of the giant-cell tumour and its so-called variants are similar to normal osteoclasts, and their identical histochemical behaviour and ultrastructural similarity indicate a close relationship; hence the use of the term "osteoclastoma" seems to be justified. Most authorities agree that the multinucleated giant cells are derived from mononuclear stromal cells, possibly of undifferentiated mesenchymal cell origin, or from cells of histiocytic macrophage origin, either by agglutination or conglomeration. Much less likely is an origin of the giant cells by mitotic division of stromal cells in the absence of cytoplasmic segmentation.

The formation of bone or osteoid tissue is occasionally seen in giant-cell tumours. It usually appears to be reactive in nature, although the possibility that the tumour cells can themselves form bone has not been completely excluded.

4 Marrow Tumours (Round-Cell Tumours)

4.1 Ewing Sarcoma (Figs. 96–103)

A malignant tumour with a rather uniform histological appearance composed of densely packed, glycogen-rich small cells with round nuclei but without prominent nucleoli or distinct cytoplasmic outlines. The tumour tissue is typically divided into irregular strands or lobules by fibrous septa, but the intercellular network of reticulin fibres, which is a feature of malignant lymphoma, is not seen. Mitoses are generally infrequent. Haemorrhage and extensive areas of necrosis are common.

The nature and origin of this tumour have been debated since Ewing (1921) described it as an "endothelial myeloma". The difficulties of differential diagnosis within the group of malignant round-cell tumours of bone, and specifically of separation between Ewing sarcoma, malignant lymphoma and metastatic neuroblastoma, are well known. The presence of intracellular glycogen in alcohol-fixed specimens and even after neutral formalin fixation aids the diagnosis of Ewing sarcoma, as glycogen is typically absent in lymphoma and most cases of neuroblastoma. The urinary excretion of catecholamines should be determined in all cases of this type, as it is increased in a high proportion of cases (approximately 80%)

of neuroblastoma. Silver stains show a lobular distribution of the reticulin fibres circumscribing large areas of tumour cells. In the zones of necrobiosis the nuclei of the tumour cells are often small and pyknotic, about the size of a lymphocyte. Pseudorosettes or tumour cells of larger size are present in some tumours, making the distinction from primitive neuroectodermal tumours of bone (PNET) difficult.

Ewing sarcoma usually occurs in patients between the ages of 5 and 15 years. The common sites are the shafts and metaphyses of long bones (femur, tibia, humerus and fibula) although some flat bones (pelvis or scapula) may also be involved. On X-ray examination the tumours are usually seen to be osteolytic but the bone destruction is often associated with patchy reactive bone formation or with periosteal bone formation, which may show a characteristic "onion-skin" appearance.

Ewing sarcoma metastasizes early, to the lungs and to other bones. The striking tendency to involve other bones has suggested a multicentric origin. Metastasis in regional lymph nodes or to the central nervous system is infrequent.

4.2 Primitive Neuroectodermal Tumour of Bone (PNET)
(Figs. 104–106)

A rare and highly malignant tumour that resembles the peripheral neuroepithelioma of soft tissues. Its distinction from Ewing sarcoma, when based solely on routine microscopy, is difficult and uncertain.

PNET is characterized histologically by the presence of numerous Homer-Wright rosettes or pseudorosettes distributed in a haphazard fashion, and by a greater degree of cellular and nuclear pleomorphism than in Ewing sarcoma. Glycogen deposits are present in about half the cases. Electron microscopy shows the presence of neurosecretory granules, intermediate filaments and neurotubule-like structures. However, unlike in metastatic neuroblastoma, urinary catecholamine excretion is negative in PNET, and this helps to distinguish these lesions.

In recent years the distinction between PNET and Ewing sarcoma has also been based particularly on the results of immunohistochemical staining with neuron-specific enolase (NSE) and other neural markers (HNK-1, HBA-71 and others). These can be expected to be positive in PNET. However, they have also been found positive in several cases in which the other histological features are those of Ewing sarcoma. Moreover, the presence of a reciprocal 11:22 chromosome translocation shared by both tumours suggests a histogenetic relationship. At present it is a matter of debate whether all Ewing sarcomas are actually PNET, or whether the diagnosis of PNET should be restricted only to atypical Ewing sarcomas displaying morphological evidence of neural differentiation.

4.3 Malignant Lymphoma of Bone (Figs. 107–110)

A malignant lymphoid tumour considered to be primary in the bone.

There can be a rather varied histological structure. The tumour cells are usually rounded and rather pleomorphic and may have well-defined cytoplasmic outlines; many of their nuclei are indented (cleaved) or horseshoe-shaped and have prominent nucleoli. In most cases numerous reticulin fibres are present and are distributed uniformly between the tumour cells.

This tumour was formerly referred to as "reticulum-cell sarcoma", first described by Parker and Jackson as a primary lesion to be regarded as distinct from Ewing sarcoma because of its characteristic histology and better prognosis. The tumour cells were then considered of histiocytic origin. Since the advent of newer classifications (Lennert, Lukes and Collins) of the non-Hodgkin lymphomas, it has been shown that the majority of "histiocytic" tumours were in fact B- or T-cell lymphomas, and that true "histiocytic" lymphomas are rare.

Although the classification of nodal lymphomas has undergone great changes, no definite and universally accepted classification scheme has been developed, particularly for the rare primary lymphomas of bone.

"Primary" lymphoma of bone is defined as a solitary osseous lesion without involvement of other osseous or nonosseous sites within 6 months on the onset of symptoms. The involvement of regional lymph nodes does not exclude the diagnosis of primary lymphoma of bone.

Given this definition it becomes evident that many of the lymphomas reported in the older literature as "primary" in bone cannot be accepted as such by present standards because they were not adequately staged. Furthermore, they did not have the benefit of the new staging procedures such as radionuclide scanning, computed tomography and magnetic resonance imaging. Most of these cases were probably secondary deposits in bone derived from tumours of lymph nodes or from other extranodal lesions, which, although morphologically indistinguishable, have a different clinical behaviour and a worse prognosis.

Malignant lymphoma of bone can occur at any age, but is most common in patients over 20 years of age, differing from Ewing sarcoma in this respect. The long bones, ilium and spine are commonly affected. The lesions are most often ill-defined, mixed lytic-blastic to purely lytic; however, sometimes there is widespread infiltration of bone without much alteration in radiographic appearance.

Histologically, all reported cases of primary lymphoma of bone are of the diffuse type. The tumour cells are generally subclassified according to nuclear size and shape as cleaved, non-cleaved or pleomorphic. The great majority are large cleaved cells. The prognosis seems to be more favourable in tumours with a predominantly cleaved cell population. Very rarely primary bone lymphomas are composed predominantly of *well-differentiated lymphocytic cells*. These must be distinguished from secondary involvement from a nodal lymphoma. In either type, primary or secondary, leukaemic changes in the peripheral blood frequently develop.

4.4 Myeloma (Figs. 111–114)

A malignant tumour, usually with multiple or diffuse bone involvement, by neoplastic plasma cells showing varying degrees of immaturity, including atypical forms. The lesions are often associated with the presence of abnormal proteins in the blood and urine, and occasionally with the presence of amyloid or para-amyloid in the tumour tissue or other organs.

Most cases of myeloma present with multiple bone lesions ("multiple myeloma", "myelomatosis"), this being one of the most frequent malignant conditions of the skeleton. It usually occurs in patients between 50 and 70 years of age; the common sites are the spine, pelvis, ribs, sternum, skull and the metaphysis of the long bones, that is, the bones that contain red marrow in the adult. The lesions appear either as focal osteolytic areas or as areas of diffuse marrow replacement without alteration in bone structure. Exceptionally, myeloma may appear as a sclerosing dense radiographic lesion, either solitary or disseminated, which is associated in about one-third of the patients with progressive peripheral neuropathy.

Abnormal values for certain laboratory tests (anaemia, increased plasma globulin, elevated erythrocyte sedimentation rate, monoclonal spike in globulin fraction of serum electrophoresis, Bence Jones proteins in the urine, hypercalcaemia) are generally diagnostic for myelomatosis. These tests are usually negative in patients with solitary myeloma.

In the later stages of the disease renal insufficiency may occur, due to deposits of Bence Jones protein in the renal tubules, nephrolithiasis secondary to massive osteolysis and hypercalcaemia and amyloidosis. This is the most serious and lethal complication.

Much more rarely, an apparently single bone lesion is found to have the histological structure of myeloma. These cases usually occur in a younger age group than multiple myeloma. A diagnosis of solitary myeloma must always be approached with caution, as the majority of cases progress to generalized myelomatosis.

Waldenström macroglobulinaemia is a rare neoplastic disease of the haematopoietic system, related to multiple myeloma, differing only in that the cells are plasmacytoid with lymphocyte-like nuclei and produce a monoclonal high molecular weight protein, the IgM macroglobulin.

5 Vascular Tumours

Vascular tumours of bone show a wide range of histological appearance, varying from well-differentiated vasoformative lesions to highly anaplastic tumours. It is sometimes difficult to make a clear distinction between the relatively common haemangiomas and the rare angiosarcomas. The existing nomenclature of malignant vascular tumours is confusing. The terms "haemangiosarcoma", "haemangioendothelioma" and "haemangioendotheliosarcoma" have been used as synonyms, and have been applied to a wide variety of malignant vascular tumours. At the same time, these entities are generally divided into different grades, from well-differentiated (grade I haemangioendothelioma) to poorly differentiated (grade III haemangioendothelioma). The rare haemangiopericytoma originating in bone is considered in all reports a distinct entity.

In view of the confusion still prevailing, the present scheme of classification separates malignant vascular lesions of bone into an intermediate or indeterminate group (essentially low-grade tumours), which includes haemangioendothelioma and the rare haemangiopericytoma, and a clearly malignant group, angiosarcoma (haemangiosarcoma). Some cases of haemangiopericytoma may present frankly malignant histological features and a metastatic potential, and are also included in the malignant group. An indisputable case of lymphangiosarcoma of bone has not yet been reported.

5.1 Benign

5.1.1 Haemangioma (Figs. 115, 116)

A benign tumour or malformation consisting of well-formed blood vessels of either a capillary or a cavernous type.

A clear distinction between some capillary haemangiomas and well-differentiated haemangioendotheliomas may sometimes be difficult. Some of these lesions are clearly malformations; others, because of their growth potential, are regarded as benign tumours. They occur most commonly in the vertebrae, often without clinical symptoms, and also in the skull, where they commonly produce a characteristic "sun-ray" radiological appearance.

Multiple haemangiomas ("systematized haemangiomatosis") of bone are encountered; they may or may not be associated with soft tissue haemangiomatosis. So-called massive osteolysis ("disappearing" or "phantom" bone disease) is a rare condition possibly related to haemangiomatosis.

5.1.2 Lymphangioma

A benign tumour or malformation consisting of lymph vessels, usually in the form of dilated cystic spaces.

These lesions are extremely rare. Virtually all cases show multiple skeletal involvement. They often occur in association with soft tissue lesions of the same type.

5.1.3 Glomus Tumour (Glomangioma)

A benign lesion consisting of uniform cells with round regular nuclei, sharply defined cell borders and pale cytoplasm, intimately associated with vascular structures and probably derived from the neuromyoarterial glomus.

The occurrence of glomus tumours of the skeleton is extremely rare, but authenticated cases have been described within a terminal phalanx. More common is the erosion of bone by a glomus tumour originating in the adjacent soft tissues.

5.2 Intermediate or Indeterminate

5.2.1 Haemangioendothelioma (Figs. 117–120)

An aggressive, but virtually nonmetastasizing tumour characterized by the presence of solid cell cords and vascular endothelial structures. The endothelial cells are often prominent and plump, but the frankly malignant histological features of angiosarcoma are lacking.

A reticulin stain is important for the recognition of this entity. Haemangioendotheliomas are rare tumours. Those with a predominance of epithelioid or histiocytoid endothelial cells have been referred to as "epithelioid haemangioendotheliomas", "histiocytoid haemangiomas" and "myxoid angioblastomas". In general, they have the same histological features as the soft tissue tumours that are referred to by the same name. They commonly recur locally after excision, but rarely metastasize. In about one-third of cases, multiple bone lesions, usually in the same extremity, may be present.

The terms "haemangioendothelioma" (graded I–III) and "haemangiosarcoma" are used interchangeably by some authors.

5.2.2 Haemangiopericytoma (Fig. 121)

An aggressive tumour characterized by a pattern of vascular spaces lined by a single layer of endothelial cells surrounded by zones of proliferating cells.

Only a small number of tumours with a histological structure similar to that of haemangiopericytoma of soft tissues have been reported in the skeleton. The exact histological criteria for the recognition of haemangiopericytoma, and for the separation of low-grade and malignant variants, have not yet been satisfactorily defined. The perivascular pattern of these tumours can best be recognized in reticulin preparation.

5.3 Malignant

5.3.1 Angiosarcoma (Figs. 122–125)

A malignant tumour characterized by the formation of irregular anastomosing vascular channels lined by one or more layers of atypical endothelial cells, often of immature appearance, and accompanied by solid masses of poorly differentiated or anaplastic tissue.

Angiosarcomas of bone are rare, and it must be emphasized that other highly vascular tumours, particularly the relatively common telangiectatic osteosarcoma, are sometimes erroneously diagnosed as angiosarcoma. A positive immunocytochemical reaction for factor VIII or for *Ulex* lectin can be useful in identifying the vascular nature of a poorly differentiated malignant tumour.

Angiosarcomas are highly malignant tumours that metastasize rapidly to the lungs. Multiple angiosarcomas of bone, or of bone and soft tissues, can occur. Synonyms include "haemangiosarcoma" and "malignant haemangioendothelioma".

5.3.2 Malignant haemangiopericytoma

Some cases of haemangiopericytoma show evident features of malignancy, frank anaplasia and metastatic potential, associated with a bad prognosis.

6 Other Connective Tissue Tumours

6.1 Benign

6.1.1 Benign Fibrous Histiocytoma

A benign lesion characterized by the presence of spindle-celled fibrous tissue with a storiform pattern and containing a variable number of multinucleated giant cells, hemosiderin pigment and lipid-bearing histiocytes (xanthoma cells).

These histological features are identical to those of metaphyseal fibrous defect (fibrous cortical defect and nonossifying fibroma). However, almost all authorities consider metaphyseal fibrous defect a non-neoplastic lesion (possibly a developmental anomaly), since it is often self-limited or may become ossified and disappear. The term "benign fibrous histiocytoma" implies a neoplasm, and its existence as a separate entity is based on clinical differences from metaphyseal fibrous defect. These clinical differences include an older age of the patients and the lesion being confined to the diaphysis or epiphysis of long bones, or to the pelvis and ribs, clavicle or spine. Moreover, the lesion is generally painful even in the absence of fracture. Some exceptional cases of atypical fibrous histiocytoma have been reported, but their histological features are not yet clearly defined.

6.1.2 Lipoma

A benign tumour of mature adipose tissue with no evidence of cellular atypia.

There are two types of lipoma, an intraosseous and a periosteal type, the latter usually inducing new bone formation. Although these lesions constitute an established entity, they are rare. They usually occur in adults, and may be mistaken for other more serious types of lesions, or may be associated with a bone infarct. A variety of skeletal sites are involved, most commonly long bones and calcaneus.

Angiolipomatous malformations, usually of the vertebral bodies, have been described, but they should be distinguished from true lipomas.

6.2 Intermediate

6.2.1 Desmoplastic Fibroma (Figs. 126–128)

A benign but locally aggressive tumour characterized by the formation of abundant collagen fibres by the tumour cells. The tissue is sparsely cellular, and the nuclei are ovoid or elongated. The cellularity, pleomorphism and mitotic activity which are features of fibrosarcoma are lacking.

The term "desmoplastic fibroma" was applied by Jaffe in 1958 to describe a group of rare fibrous tissue lesions in bone, distinct from fibrosarcoma on the one hand and from various benign lesions on the other, presenting often a locally aggressive behaviour. Histologically, the lesions resemble "desmoid tumours" of soft tissues. The tumours usually occur in adolescents or young adults and involve a variety of skeletal sites, including long bones, vertebrae and pelvis. Local recurrence sometimes follows excision, but no metastases have been reported. The distinction between desmoplastic fibroma and well-differentiated fibrosarcoma is often difficult.

A small lesion originating beneath the periosteum and eroding the underlying cortex is referred to as a "periosteal desmoid", which though considered to be a periosteal variant of desmoplastic fibroma, is a reactive rather than a neoplastic lesion.

6.3 Malignant

6.3.1 Fibrosarcoma (Figs. 129–131)

A malignant tumour characterized by the formation by the tumour cells of interlacing bundles of collagen fibres, and by the absence of other types of histological differentiation, such as cartilage or bone.

Fibrosarcomas of bone were originally classified with osteosarcomas, but the view that they should be regarded as a separate group has become generally accepted.

Fibrosarcomas usually involve long bones, particularly the lower part of the femur and the upper part of the tibia. They occur in older patients than do osteosarcomas, mostly in persons from 20 to 60 years of age. Radiologically, they appear as osteolytic, poorly defined lesions. Fibrosarcomas are a variable group as far as their histological structure is concerned. Some are highly differentiated, rich in collagen, and show only slight mitotic activity or cellular pleomorphism, while others are relatively undifferentiated. There is some evidence that the highly differentiated tumours have a better prognosis than the others.

It may be difficult, particularly in limited biopsy specimens, to distinguish between poorly differentiated fibrosarcomas, osteosarcomas containing only a small amount of tumour bone, and poorly differentiated or undifferentiated tumours of other types. Similarly, it may be difficult with a limited sample of tissue to distinguish a highly differentiated fibrosarcoma from a desmoplastic fibroma. Many cases formerly classified as pleomorphic fibrosarcoma are at present referred to as "malignant fibrous histiocytoma".

6.3.2 Malignant Fibrous Histiocytoma (Figs. 132–135)

A rather infrequent highly malignant tumour of bone with the same variable structure as the more common tumour of soft tissue. It is characterized histologically by bundles of collagen fibres and spindle-shaped fibroblast-like cells arranged in a storiform or "cartwheel" pattern together with rounded cells showing features of histiocytes. The latter have ovoid, indented nuclei and cytoplasm with phagocytic activity and can transform into foam cells. The tumours frequently contain cells with bizarre, pleomorphic and multiple nuclei. Typical multinucleated giant cells of osteoclastic type as well as atypical ones are often found. Mitotic activity and cellular atypia are common. Relatively conspicuous inflammatory cells, predominantly lymphocytes, are characteristic.

Radiographs show a radiolucent lesion with poorly defined permeative margins destroying the cortex and often extensively invading extraosseous soft tissues. Malignant fibrous histiocytoma usually occurs in adults and commonly involves the long bones, predominantly the metaphyseal region of the femur or the tibia. An association with bone infarct is not infrequent, and a possible aetiologic relationship has been suggested. Some authors accept the presence of infrequent areas of bone or cartilage as consistent with the diagnosis of malignant fibrous histiocytoma, but this is not accepted by others, who classify such a lesion as osteosarcoma with a predominant fibrohistiocytic pattern.

Malignant fibrous histiocytoma of bone seems to be overdiagnosed. A wide biopsy or thorough study of the operative specimen is often necessary. Immunohistochemical studies and electron microscopy may be helpful by excluding other lines of specific differentiation.

6.3.3 Liposarcoma

A malignant tumour characterized by lipoblastic differentiation, as shown by the presence of atypical lipoblasts.

This is an exceedingly rare type of bone tumour, although authenticated cases have been reported. They almost invariably occur in long bones, usually in tibia and femur.

6.3.4 Malignant Mesenchymoma (Figs. 136–138)

A malignant tumour characterized by the presence of multiple types of connective tissue differentiation, particularly those not usually encountered in the skeleton.

This is an exceedingly rare type of tumour and needs further study. The few reported cases show a combination of osteosarcomatous and liposarcomatous components. These tumours have been referred to as "primary osteoliposarcoma of bone".

6.3.5 Leiomyosarcoma

A rare malignant tumour characterized by intersecting bundles of spindle-shaped cells with elongated, blunt-ended, central nuclei and scant fibrillar cytoplasm, resembling smooth muscle differentiation. There are variable degrees of nuclear atypia and pleomorphism, with the presence of hyperchromatic or bizarre nuclei and generally infrequent mitotic activity. The stroma varies from areas with scarce fibres to broad hyalinized fibrous zones.

Leiomyosarcoma of bone is more common in elderly patients and involves predominantly long tubular bones, especially the femur and tibia, about the knee.

Radiographically, leiomyosarcoma appears as an ill-defined osteolytic lesion, with features very similar to those of fibrosarcoma. Electron microscopy and immunohistochemical studies with smooth muscle markers (actin and desmin) aid in diagnosis and separation from fibrosarcoma.

The course of osseous leiomyosarcoma is variable and seems related to the grade of histological differentiation.

6.3.6 Undifferentiated Sarcoma (Fig. 139)

A malignant tumour with a pleomorphic spindle-celled structure but devoid of any specific pattern of histological differentiation.

In a limited biopsy specimen, a poorly differentiated fibrosarcoma, an osteosarcoma with relatively little tumour bone, a lymphoma, or even an undifferentiated metastatic carcinoma can pose practical difficulties of identification and thus be confused with cases properly belonging to this group. Even after the study of adequate samples of tissue, including cytomorphological and immunohistochemical methods, and subsequent follow-up investigation, rare cases remain in which the tumour is regarded as primary in bone but where no specific pattern of differentiation can be detected. Consequently, this group is regarded as an essential part of the classification.

7 Other Tumours

7.1 Chordoma (Figs. 140–143)

A locally aggressive or malignant tumour characterized by a lobular arrangement of tissue, which is usually made up of cords and sheets of highly vacuolated cells ("physaliphorous cells") and mucoid intercellular material.

These tumours are almost always restricted to the axial skeleton; this, together with their histological structure, suggests that they originate from notochordal tissue. Although often regarded as arising from developmental remnants of notochord, chordomas are usually found in patients over 40 years of age. Men are more commonly affected than women. The sacral and spheno-occipital regions are the commonest sites. The intervening vertebrae are involved only rarely. Half the vertebral lesions occur in the cervical spine.

Chordomas are slowly growing tumours. They infiltrate adjacent structures and recur after local resection. Although these tumours almost invariably prove fatal, metastases develop rarely and then usually at a late stage after many attempts at local surgical treatment.

The histological distinction between chordoma and chondrosarcoma is sometimes difficult. Some chordomas of the spheno-occipital region contain more or less extensive chondrosarcoma-like areas, and are known as "chondroid chordomas". The positive immunocytochemical reaction for cytokeratin identifies them as chordomas, chondroid variant. A mucin-secreting carcinoma may mimic the histological appearance of chordoma, but the cells of a chordoma contain glycogen and not mucin. Some chordomas have a more cellular and pleomorphic histological structure than others, but this pattern does not appear to show any clear correlation with either rate of growth or frequency of metastasis. However, it seems that the chondroid chordomas have a much better prognosis than classic chordomas.

7.2 Adamantinoma of Long Bones (Figs. 144–146)

A malignant, or at least locally aggressive, tumour characterized by a wide range of morphological patterns, most commonly the presence of circumscribed masses or tubular formation of apparently epithelial cells surrounded by spindle-celled fibrous tissue.

This is a well-established but rare tumour that almost invariably involves the shaft of the tibia at its anterior aspect. Radiographs show a lucent, frequently multilocular lesion with sclerotic borders. It usually occurs in adults, although it seems not to be as rare in children under 10 years of age as was formerly reported. The peripheral cells of the supposed epithelial formations are columnar and palisaded, while the central cells have a stellate arrangement and are separated by spaces; this gives the lesion some degree of resemblance to the ameloblastoma ("adamantinoma") of the jaw, and to other epithelial tumours of the basal-cell type.

The histogenesis is uncertain. The histological similarity to ameloblastoma has suggested an epithelial origin, despite the paradox of the intraosseous situation of the tumours, and this appears to be confirmed by the results of electron microscopy and of immunohistochemical studies (keratin positive and factor VIII negative).

Not infrequently, adamantinoma may be associated with or mimic fibrous dysplasia or osteofibrous dysplasia, and this has suggested a close relationship between these entities.

7.3 Neurilemoma

A benign tumour of nerve sheath origin, having the same morphological features as soft tissue neurilemomas, but originating within a bone.

Intraosseous neurilemomas are very rare, but a small number of authenticated cases, most frequently involving mandible and sacrum and presumably arising from intraosseous nerves, have been reported.

7.4 Neurofibroma

A benign neurogenic tumour of Schwann cells and fibroblasts having the same morphological features as soft tissue neurofibromas, but originating within a bone.

It is composed of spindle-shaped or stellate cells with elongated wavy nuclei. The stroma is oedematous with diffusely distributed collagen fibres. Occasionally, cells with large pleomorphic nuclei are present, but mitotic activity is absent.

Benign nerve sheath tumours associated with von Recklinghausen disease are almost always neurofibromas. Only a few cases of intraosseous neurofibroma appear to have been authenticated, although the term is more frequently used in the radiological literature. It is well known, of course, that other types of skeletal change, including scoliosis, growth disorders, congenital bowing and pseudarthrosis, commonly occur in neurofibromatosis, but these are not associated with the presence of neurofibromatous tissue actually within the involved bones. Similarly, no cases of intraosseous malignant neurogenic tumours ("malignant schwannoma", "neurosarcoma") have been authenticated.

8 Unclassified Tumours

Any large series of bone tumours includes lesions for which a specific classification is not possible, either because the lesions in question show features that apparently belong to more than one group or because they show features that have hitherto been unrecognized. These cases, which make up a diverse group and include both benign and malignant tumours, are regarded as unclassifiable. It is hoped, of course, that further study and experience will ultimately result in their more precise recognition and classification.

9 Tumour-like Lesions

9.1 Solitary Bone Cyst (Simple or Unicameral Bone Cyst)
(Figs. 147, 148)

A unicameral cavity filled with clear or sanguineous fluid and lined by a membrane of variable thickness, which consists of loose vascular connective tissue showing scattered osteoclast giant cells and sometimes areas of recent or old haemorrhage or cholesterol clefts.

Solitary bone cysts are most frequently located in the metaphyses at the upper end of the humerus and the femur; they occur in children and adolescents. Bands or masses of fibrin-like material resembling odontogenic cementum, or of hyalinized or calcified connective tissue, are commonly present in the tissue of the wall, and occasional bone trabeculae may also be present. The gross and microscopic features are often modified by fracture. Based on the similarity between the bone cyst fluid and serum a transitory circulatory disturbance due to a developmental venous anomaly has been proposed as aetiology.

9.2 Aneurysmal Bone Cyst (Figs. 149, 150)

An expanding osteolytic lesion consisting of blood-filled spaces of variable size separated by connective tissue septa containing trabeculae of bone or osteoid tissue and osteoclast giant cells.

Prior to its recognition by Jaffe in 1950 and by Lichtenstein in 1950, examples of aneurysmal bone cyst were usually regarded as giant-cell tumours or telangiectatic osteosarcomas. It has been accepted as an entity, although in some cases its histological distinction from giant-cell tumour may be difficult or even impossible.

Aneurysmal bone cysts are usually seen in patients under 30 years of age and involve either the shafts of long bones or the vertebral column, generally arising in the posterior osseous elements. They often have an eccentric location, which, with the "ballooned-out" distension of the periosteum, was responsible for their name. Their rapid development and large size may suggest a malignant lesion, but in fact they are benign.

Cystic changes, apparently secondary and closely resembling those of aneurysmal bone cyst, are sometimes present in benign chondroblastoma, giant-cell tumour, osteoblastomas, osteosarcoma and other lesions and may involve substantial areas of tissue.

9.3 Juxta-articular Bone Cyst (Intraosseous Ganglion)
(Figs. 151, 152)

A benign, cystic, and often multiloculated lesion, made up of fibrous tissue, with extensive mucoid change, situated in the subchondral bone adjacent to a joint.

The juxta-articular bone cyst is a fairly common lesion, occurring in patients of middle age. It usually involves the bones adjacent to the hip joint, knee joint, ankle and carpal bones. In radiographs, it appears as a well-defined osteolytic area with a surrounding zone of sclerosis. It has been described as a "synovial cyst", but it lacks a synovial lining; the histological structure resembles that of a soft tissue ganglion. Similar cysts occur in osteoarthritis, and more rarely in rheumatoid arthritis.

9.4 Metaphyseal Fibrous Defect (Nonossifying Fibroma)
(Figs. 153, 154)

A well-defined, benign, non-neoplastic bone lesion, characterized by essentially the same histological features described in benign fibrous histiocytoma, that is, spindle-celled fibrous tissue with a storiform pattern and containing a variable number of multinucleated giant cells, hemosiderin pigment and lipid-bearing histiocytes (xanthoma cells).

The term "metaphyseal fibrous defect" has been used for many years and is purely descriptive and noncommittal with respect to its histogenesis. Lesions of this type are also referred to as "fibrous cortical defects", "nonossifiying fibroma", "fibrous xanthoma" or "histiocytic xanthogranuloma".

The lesions usually involve the metaphyseal region of long bones in children or adolescents, most commonly at the lower end of the femur or the upper or lower end of the tibia. The fibrous cortical defect is a fairly common, small lytic intracortical lesion of children which often disappears in a few years or may progress occasionally, extending to the medullary cavity, representing the typical features of nonossifying fibroma. It is characterized as an eccentric, sharply outlined, osteolytic defect surrounded by a thin shell of reactive bone. As growth proceeds it becomes progressively more separated from the growth plate. It is usually symptomless and in some cases may ultimately disappear. It may become painful only after a pathological fracture or when it occasionally shows a progressive, conspicuous enlargement.

Metaphyseal fibrous defect may involve multiple bones and on rare occasions present extraskeletal anomalies (Jaffe-Campanacci syndrome).

9.5 Eosinophilic Granuloma (Histiocytosis X, Langerhans Cell Granulomatosis) (Figs. 155, 156)

A non-neoplastic lesion of unknown aetiology, characterized by an intense proliferation of histiocytes with varying numbers of eosinophilic leucocytes, neutrophilic leucocytes, lymphocytes, plasma cells and multinucleate giant cells. Zones of necrosis are frequent, as is the presence of lipid-bearing foam cells, especially in multiple and older lesions.

Either solitary or multiple lesions may occur, the latter as part of the Hand-Schüller-Christian syndrome or of Letterer-Siwe disease. These all seem to be manifestations of the same basic disorder, which is sometimes referred to as "histiocytosis X" or "reticuloendotheliosis". The histiocytes have indented or lobulated nuclei, often with longitudinal grooves and abundant eosinophilic cytoplasm that contains S-100 protein. The cells frequently contain cytoplasmic inclusions called "Bierbeck granules", shaped like tennis rackets. They are characteristic of the Langerhans cells of the epidermis, and some authors use the term "Langerhans histiocytosis or granuloma" for histiocytosis X. Children and adolescents are usually involved, and common sites for bone lesions in eosinophilic granuloma include the skull, mandible, ribs, femur, vertebrae and flat bones. The lesions are osteolytic, and may be associated with periosteal reaction. Radiological distinction from Ewing sarcoma or osteomyelitis is sometimes difficult.

When large numbers of eosinophilic leucocytes are present, the histological diagnosis is usually obvious. Occasionally, however, particularly when eosinophils are relatively infrequent and histiocytic cells predominate, the histological appearance may resemble that of Hodgkin disease or even of non-Hodgkin lymphoma.

9.6 Fibrous Dysplasia and Osteofibrous Dysplasia

9.6.1 Fibrous Dysplasia (Figs. 157, 158)

A benign lesion, presumably developmental in nature, characterized by the presence of fibrous connective tissue with a characteristic whorled pattern and containing trabeculae of immature nonlamellar (woven) bone, typically not lined by osteoblasts.

Lesions of fibrous dysplasia may be solitary (monostotic) or multiple (polyostotic). The latter are occasionally accompanied by cutaneous pigmentation and, in females, by precocious puberty (Albright syndrome). Cartilage may be rarely present in solitary and more frequently in multiple lesions. Rare solitary lesions with considerable amounts of cartilage are referred to as "fibrocartilaginous dysplasia".

Fibrous dysplasia usually presents clinically during childhood or adolescence. Bones commonly involved include the femur, tibia, facial skeleton and ribs. Radiographically, the lesions often have a characteristic "ground glass" appearance. Malignant change has been reported in fibrous dysplasia, but is very rare.

9.6.2 Osteofibrous Dysplasia (Figs. 159, 160)

A rare benign lesion, almost exclusively localized in the tibia and fibula of young children. As in fibrous dysplasia the lesions are characterized by the presence of fibrous connective tissue and trabeculae of immature nonlamellar bone. In contrast to fibrous dysplasia, the surfaces of the bone trabeculae are usually covered by rows of active osteoblasts.

The term "osteofibrous dysplasia" was introduced by Campanacci in 1976, replacing the designation "ossifying fibroma" which had been used by Kempson in 1966 to describe these lesions in analogy to the process in maxillary bones, which presents similar histological features. Osteofibrous dysplasia involves predominantly the cortex of the tibia, showing a characteristic radiological loculated to bubbly appearance, with bowing of the anterior cortex. Some authors refer to this lesion as "cortical fibrous dysplasia", a more active or aggressive type of an otherwise typical fibrous dysplasia.

9.7 Myositis Ossificans (Heterotopic Ossification)
(Figs. 161, 162)

A non-neoplastic lesion, sometimes associated with trauma, characterized by proliferation of fibrous tissue and by formation of large amounts of new bone. Cartilage may also be present. The lesions may occur on the external surface of a bone or in soft tissues at a distance from the periosteal surface.

The abnormal tissue may be highly cellular. When the lesion involves the external surface of a bone, the radiological and histological distinction from juxtacortical osteosarcoma may be difficult. In the soft tissues, distinction from the rare osteosarcoma of soft tissues may also present problems, although in myositis ossificans the maturation of the abnormal tissue characteristically results in a peripheral shell of mature bone surrounding a central mass of more cellular tissue. Muscle is not necessarily involved. The lesion is not inflammatory in nature, but the term myositis ossificans is retained as it is widely used. The designation heterotopic ossification has been proposed because of its wider application to traumatic and nontraumatic lesions. Some lesions occurring on the surface of bone are referred to as "periostitis ossificans" or "reactive periostitis" and those occurring in soft tissues are at times referred to as "pseudomalignant osseous tumours of soft tissues". These local lesions must be distinguished from the rare generalized condition myositis ossificans progressiva. Periostitis ossificans is the periosteal equivalent of myositis ossificans with clinicopathological features similar to myositis ossificans or of fracture callus.

9.8 Brown Tumour of Hyperparathyroidism (Figs. 163, 164)

A circumscribed non-neoplastic lesion characterized by the presence of large numbers of osteoclast giant cells, usually arranged in groups and separated by richly vascularized fibrous tissue with areas of new bone and osteoid formation. The surrounding bone tissue frequently shows evidence of increased osteoclastic resorption. Areas of recent and old haemorrhage are common.

The brown tumour of hyperparathyroidism is easily confused with giant-cell tumour, although the typical spindle-shaped mononuclear cells of a giant-cell tumour are not usually present and the tissue is often more fibrous. The distinction between the two types of lesions is aided by their different skeletal distribution: in long bones, lesions of hyperparathyroidism usually involve the shafts, and not the ends of the bone as in giant-cell tumour. The presence of radiological and biochemical evidence of hyperparathyroidism is also important in making the diagnosis. In the jaw bones, the brown tumour of hyperparathyroidism may be histologically indistinguishable from giant-cell granuloma.

9.9 Intraosseous Epidermoid Cyst (Fig. 165)

A relatively infrequent non-neoplastic lesion, also called "keratin or squamous-epithelial cyst", which involves the jaws, the distal phalanges and the skull. It is characterized histologically by a membrane consisting of squamous epithelium, covered by laminated masses of keratin that may occupy part of the cavity.

The great majority occur in males between 20 and 50 years of age. The phalangeal lesions are most frequent in manual workers: their appearance following trauma is strong evidence for a traumatic aetiology.

Epidermoid cysts involving the skull, also referred to as "cholesteatoma", are less frequent and radiographically show a radiolucent appearance, as do the phalangeal cysts, with sharply demarcated, often slightly sclerotic margins. The aetiology is probably a developmental defect, rather than post-traumatic.

9.10 Giant-Cell (Reparative) Granuloma (Fig. 166)

An uncommon non-neoplastic lesion distinct from true giant-cell tumour, characterized histologically by a prominent fibrous stroma with areas of haemorrhage and nests of multinucleated giant cells. The giant cells are smaller than those of true giant-cell tumours. These lesions are histologically indistinguishable from the similar lesions ("brown tumour") in hyperparathyroidism. Conspicuous new bone formation is common.

Giant-cell (reparative) granuloma involves primarily the jaw bone but also the tubular bones of hands and feet, and exceptionally carpal, tarsal and other bones.

The adjective "reparative" has been dropped by many authors, because a history of trauma is infrequent. Giant-cell granulomas of hands and feet, sometimes referred to as "giant-cell reactions", occur more commonly in males, at ages ranging widely from 6 to 53 years. Radiographically, the lesions are osteolytic and trabeculated, slightly expanding the thinned cortex and commonly involving the diaphysis and metaphysis.

Unless otherwise stated, all the preparations shown in the photomicrographs reproduced on the following pages were stained with haematoxylin-eosin.

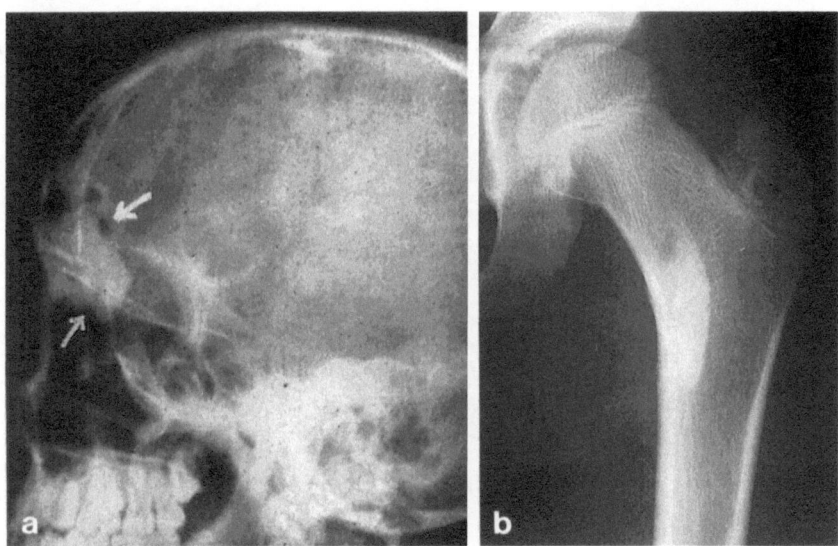

Fig. 1 a,b. *Osteoma.* **a** Male, 36 years. Frontal sinus. Radiograph. **b** Female, 9 years. Medullary tumour, upper third femur. Radiograph

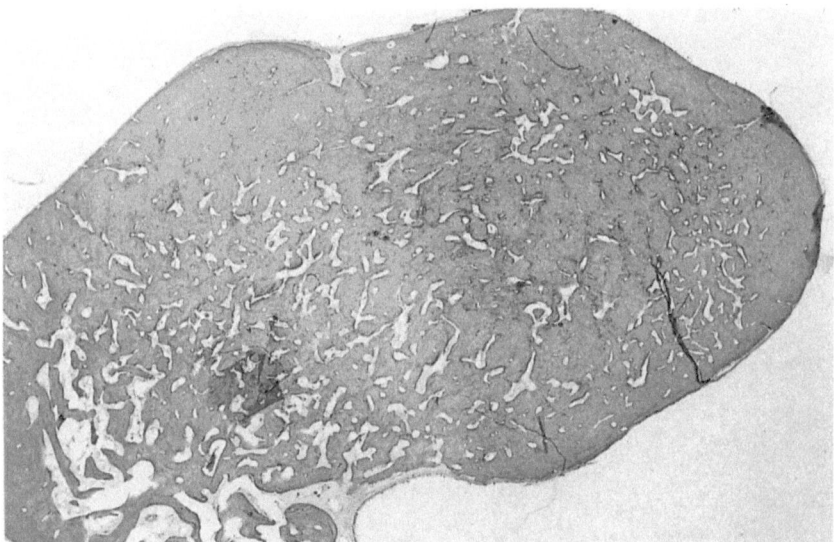

Fig. 2. *Osteoma.* Frontal sinus

44

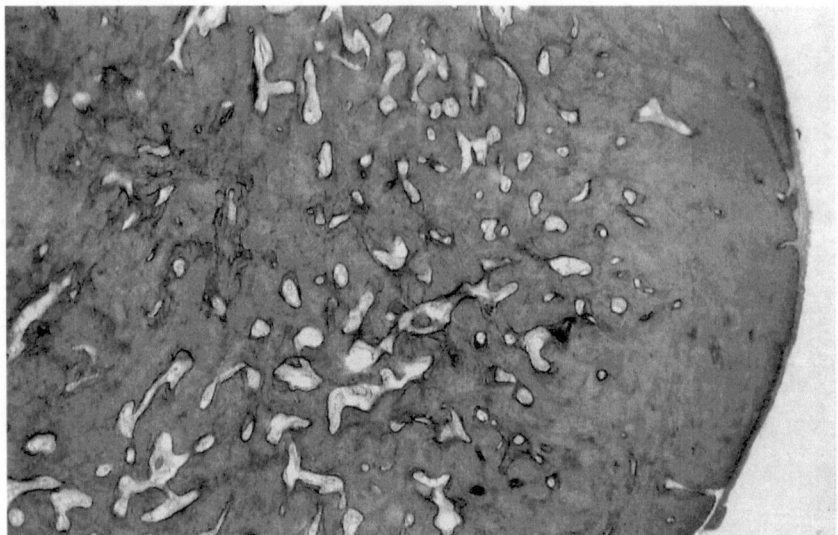

Fig. 3. *Osteoma.* Same case as in Fig. 2

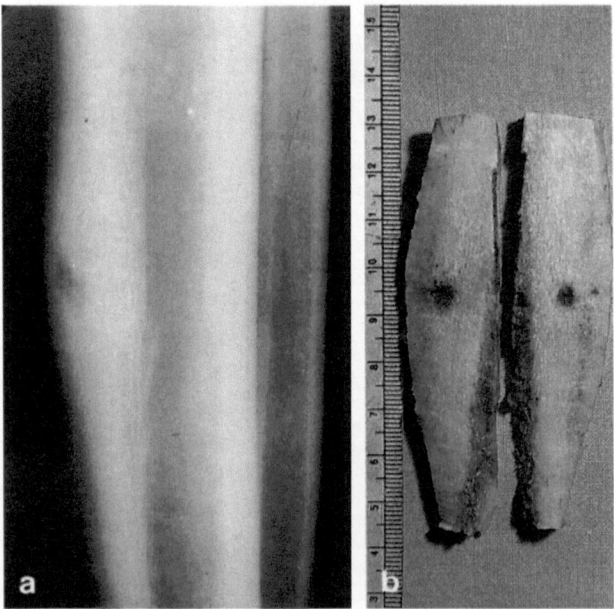

Fig. 4a, b. *Osteoid osteoma.* Male, 18 years. Shaft of tibia **a** Radiograph. **b** Photograph of specimen

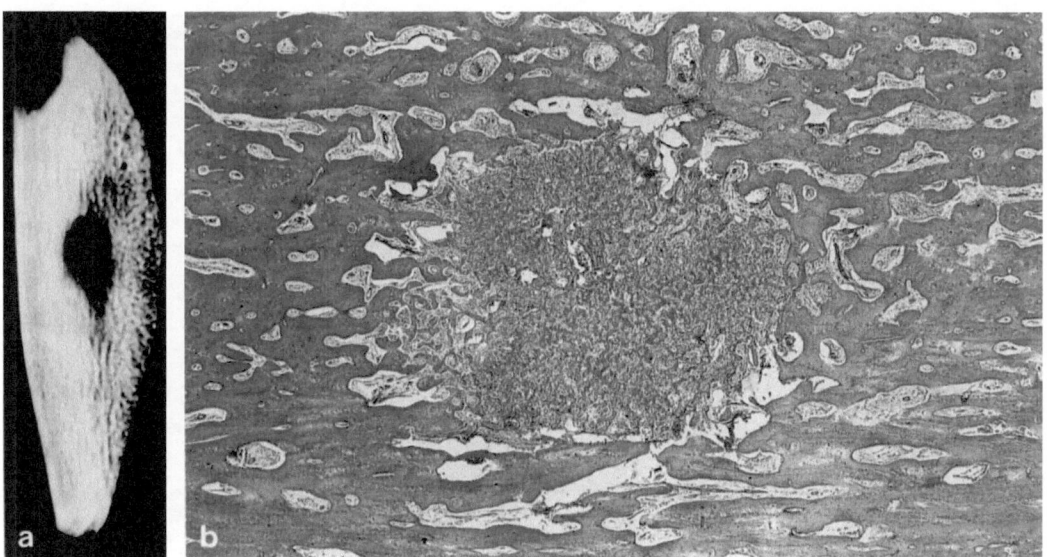

Fig. 5 a, b. *Osteoid osteoma.* **a** Radiograph of specimen of tibia. **b** Same case as **a**

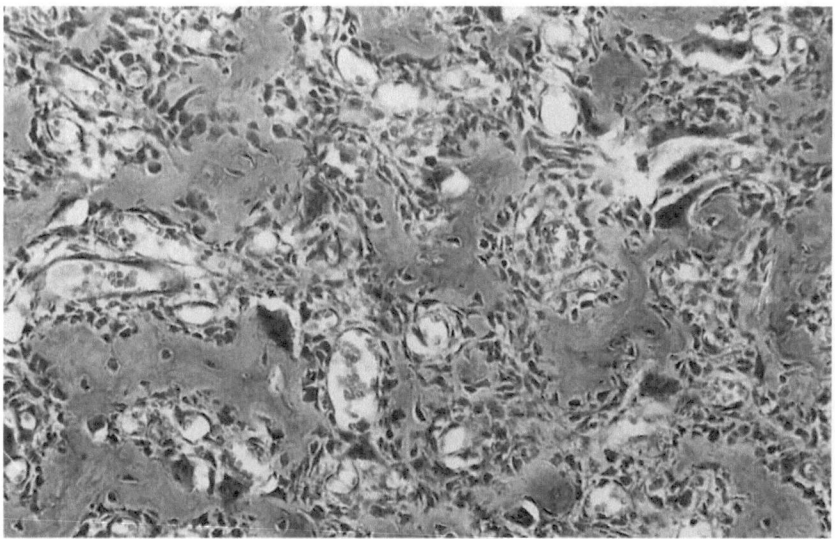

Fig. 6. *Osteoid osteoma.* Same case as Fig. 5

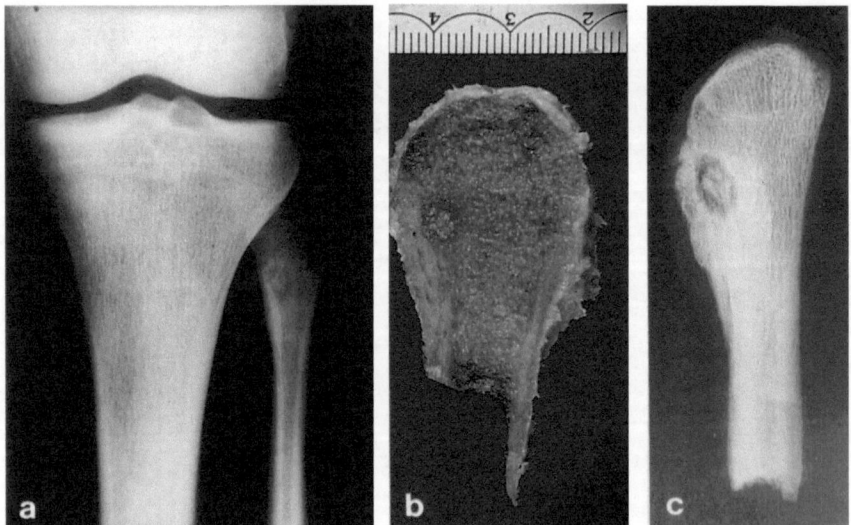

Fig. 7 a–c. *Osteoid osteoma.* Female, 15 years. Upper end of fibula. **a** Radio-graph. **b** Photograph of specimen. **c** Radiograph of specimen

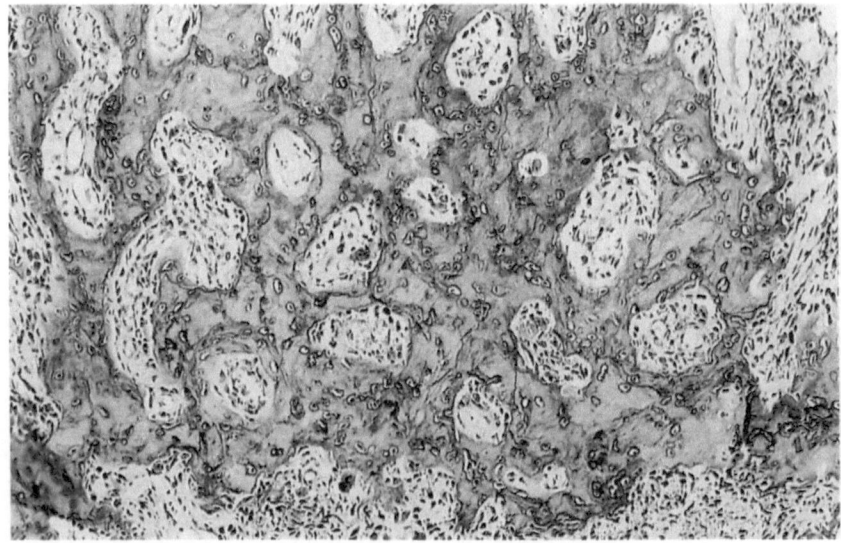

Fig. 8. *Osteoid osteoma.* Same case as Fig. 7. Calcified central zone of nidus

47

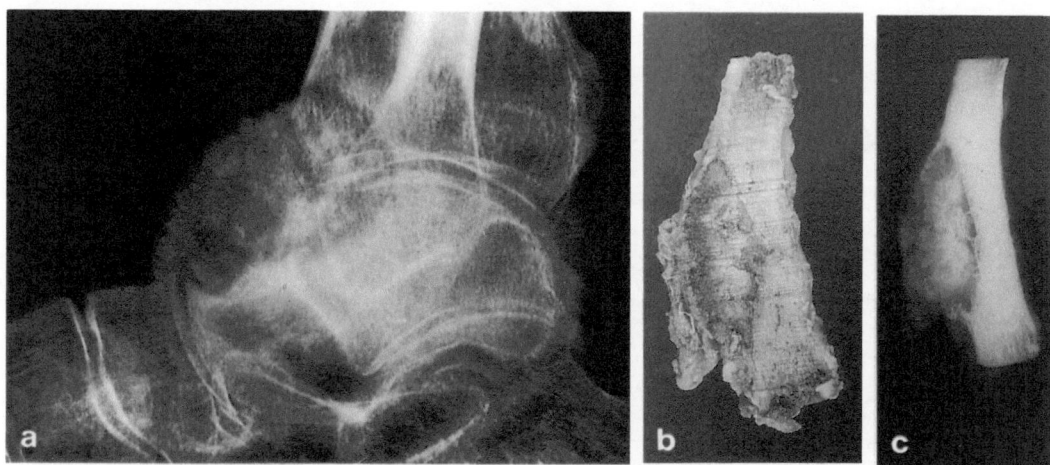

Fig. 9 a–c. *Osteoblastoma.* **a** Male, 29 years. Talus. Radiograph. **b, c** Female,
23 years. Ninth rib **b** Photograph of specimen. **c** Radiograph of specimen

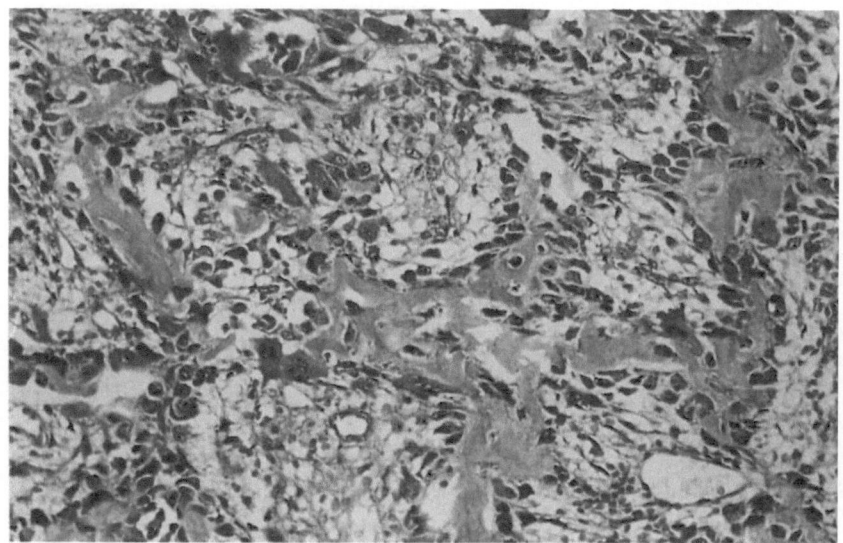

Fig. 10. *Osteoblastoma.* Same case as Fig. 9 b

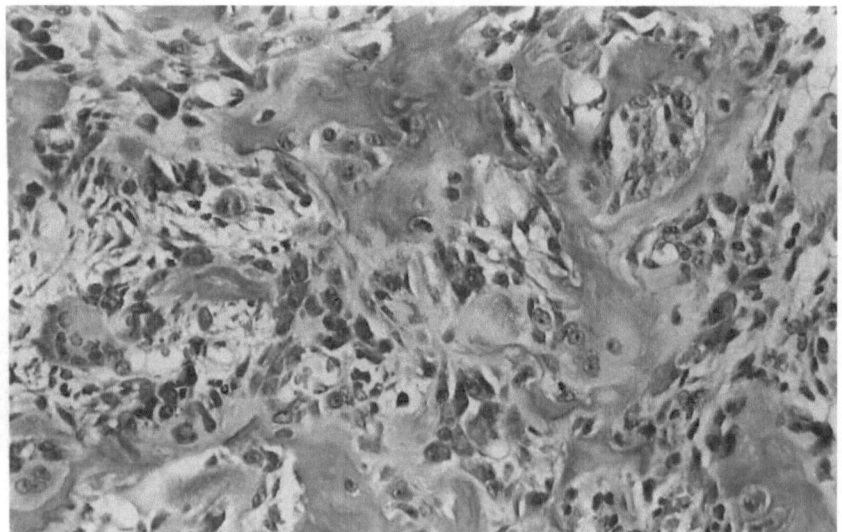

Fig. 11. *Osteoblastoma.* Same case as Fig. 9b. Bizarre area

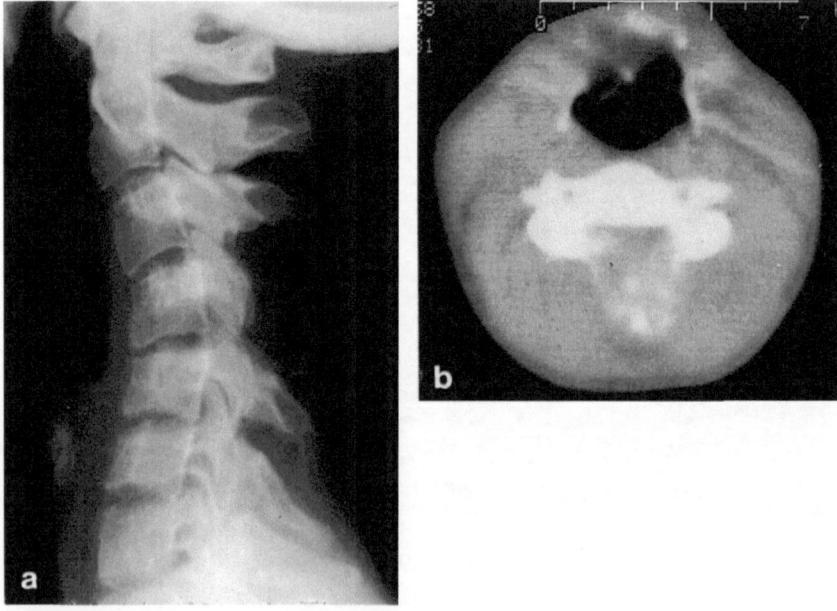

Fig. 12 a, b. *Aggressive (malignant) osteoblastoma.* Female, 19 years. Cervical spine, apophysis of fourth vertebra **a** Radiograph **b** Tomogram

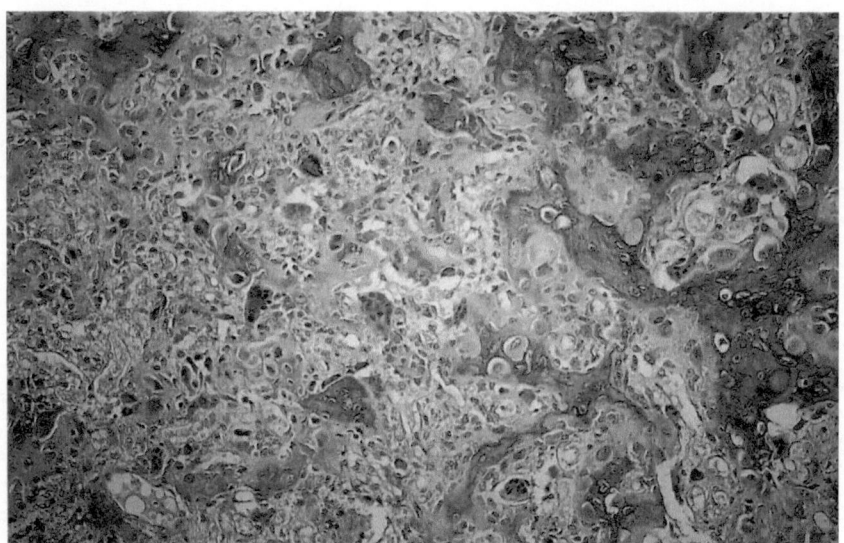

Fig. 13. *Aggressive (malignant) osteoblastoma.* Same case as Fig. 12

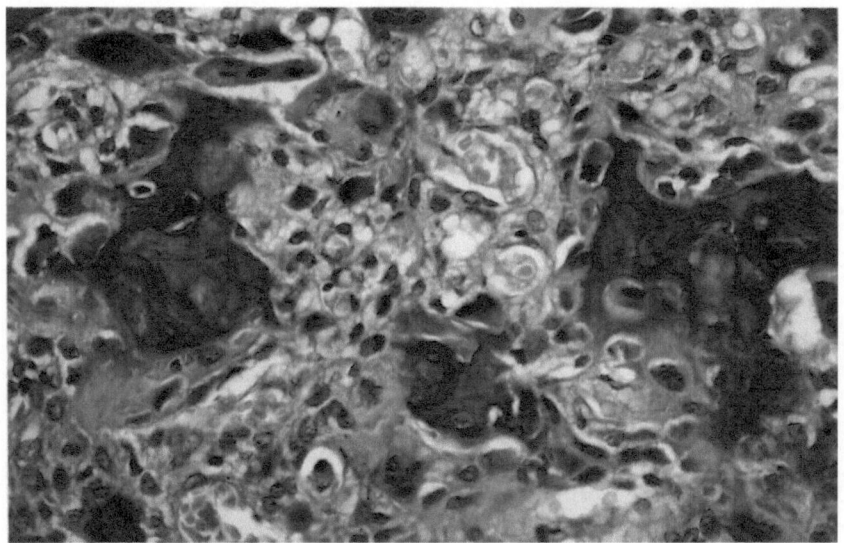

Fig. 14. *Aggressive (malignant) osteoblastoma.* Same case as Fig. 12

50

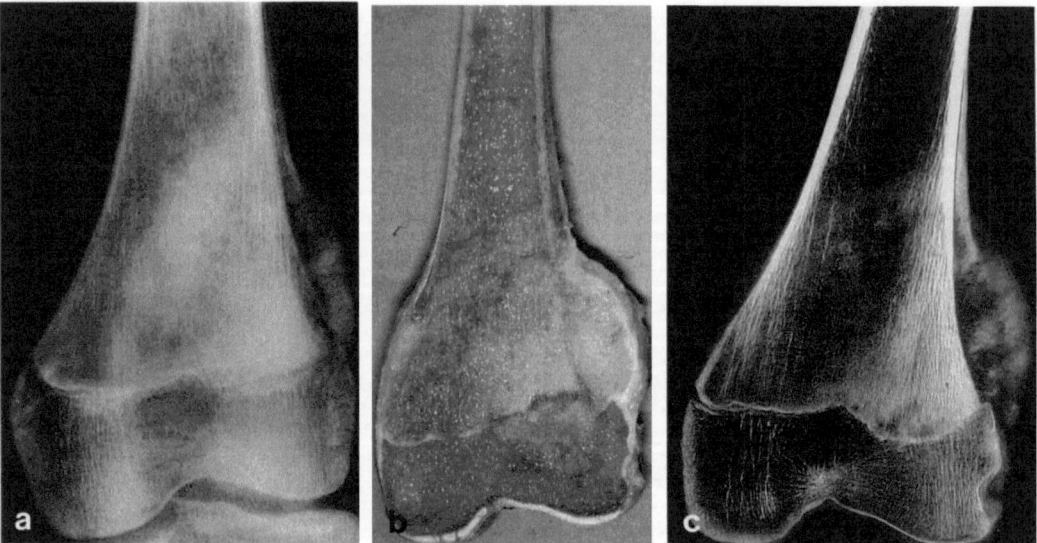

Fig. 15 a–c. *Central (medullary) osteosarcoma.* Male, 13 years. Lower metaphysis of femur **a** Radiograph. **b** Photograph of specimen. **c** Radiograph of specimen

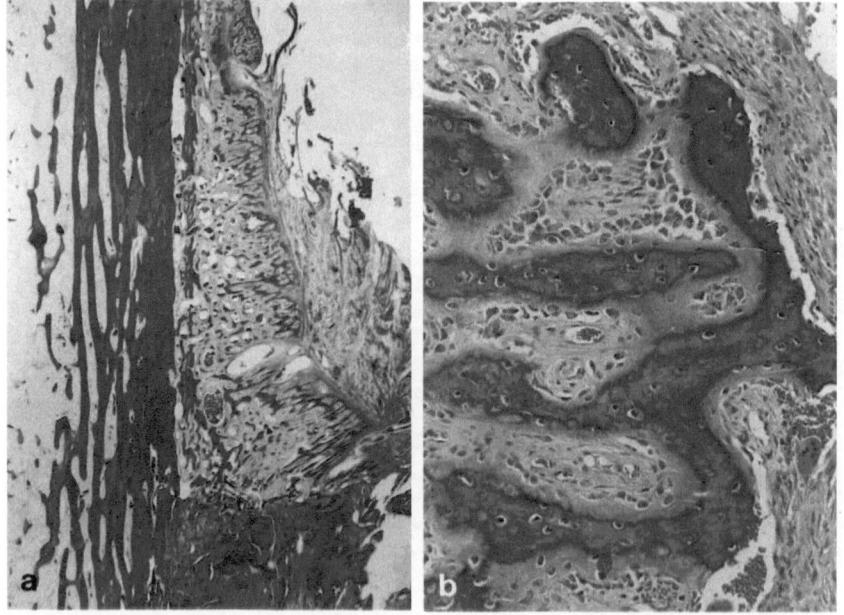

Fig. 16 a, b. *Central (medullary) osteosarcoma.* **a** Same case as Fig. 15. Periosteal reaction (Codman triangle). **b** Same case as Fig. 15. Reactive bone formation

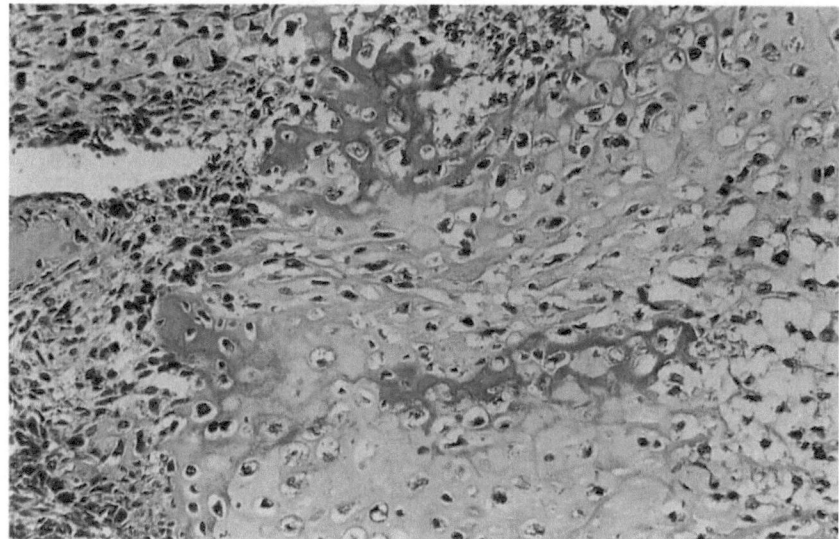

Fig. 17. *Central (medullary) osteosarcoma.* Same case as Fig. 15. Tumour bone and cartilage

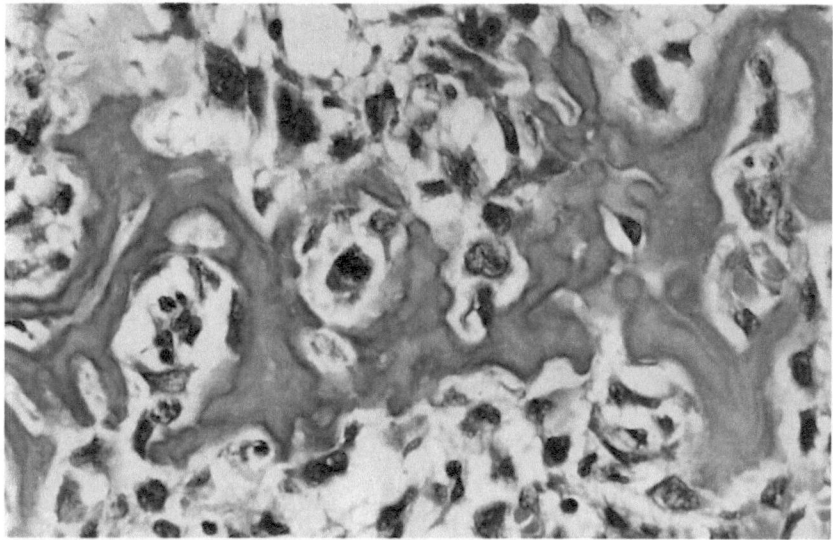

Fig. 18. *Central (medullary) osteosarcoma.* Same case as Fig. 15. Tumour bone

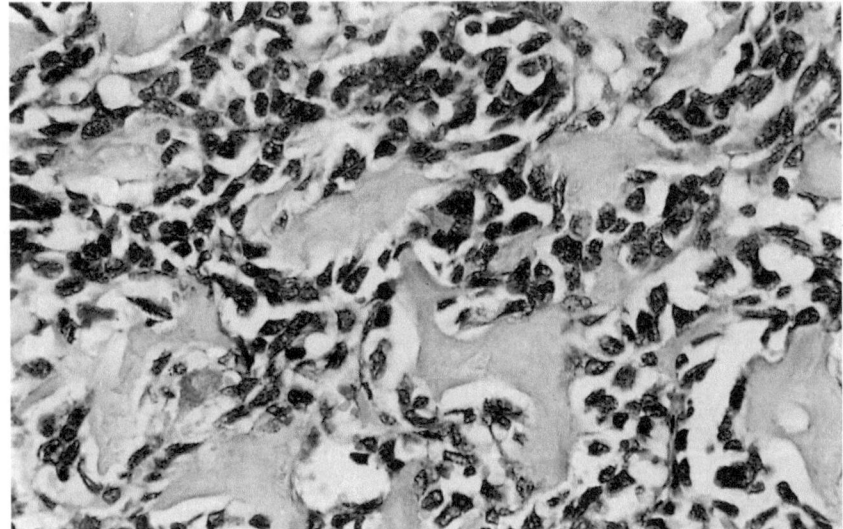

Fig. 19. *Central (medullary) osteosarcoma.* Tumour osteoid

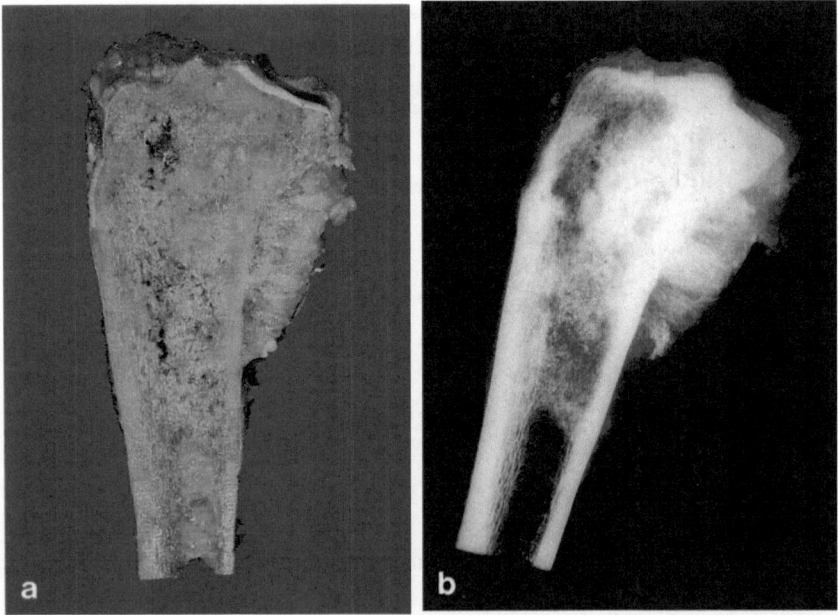

Fig. 20 a, b. *Central (medullary) osteosarcoma.* Male, 21 years. Upper end of tibia. **a** Photograph of specimen. **b** Radiograph of specimen

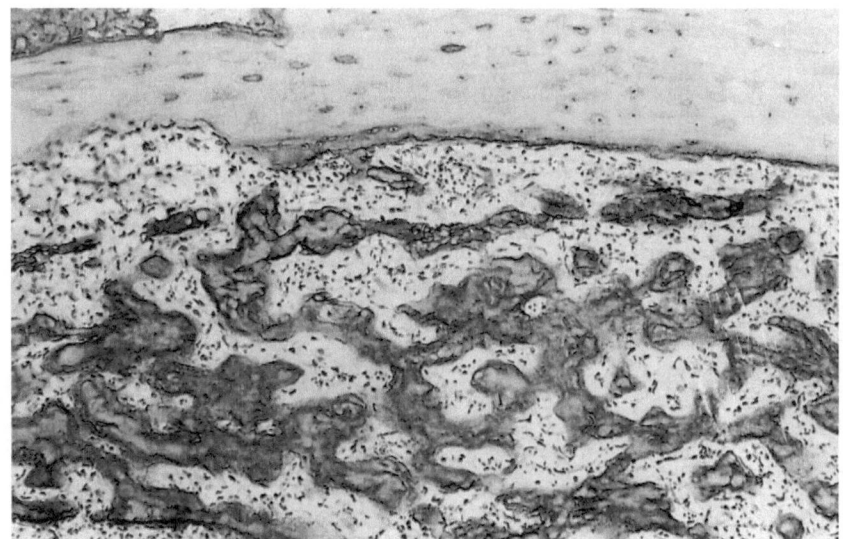

Fig. 21. *Central (medullary) osteosarcoma.* Sclerosing pattern

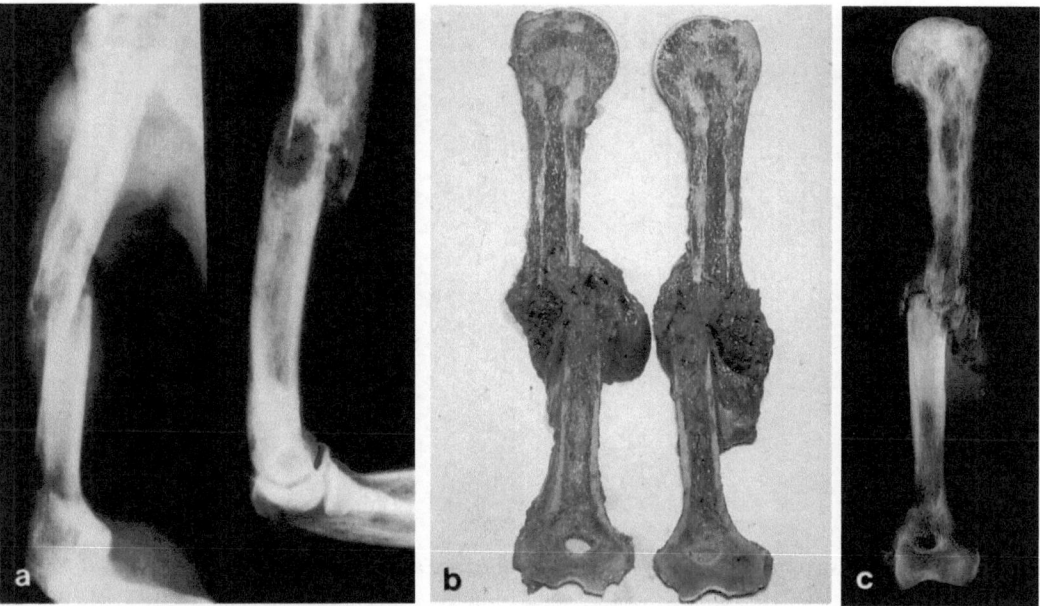

Fig. 22 a–c. *Osteosarcoma in Paget disease.* Male, 71 years. Shaft of humerus.
a Radiographs. **b** Photograph of specimen. **c** Radiograph of specimen

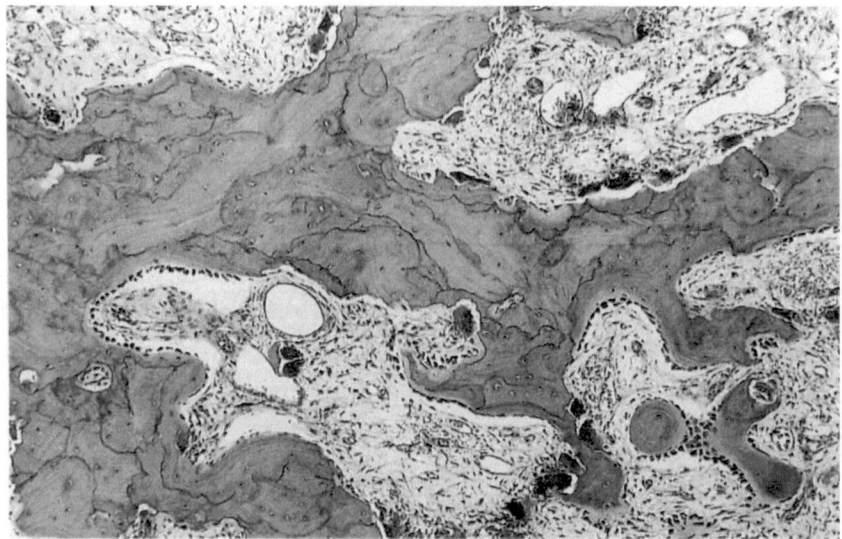

Fig. 23. *Paget disease.* Same case as Fig. 22

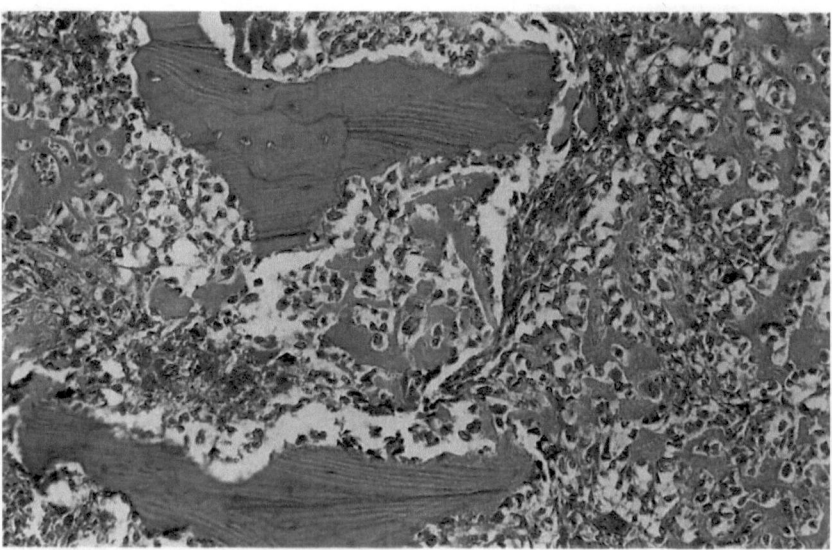

Fig. 24. *Osteosarcoma in Paget disease.* Same case as Fig. 22

55

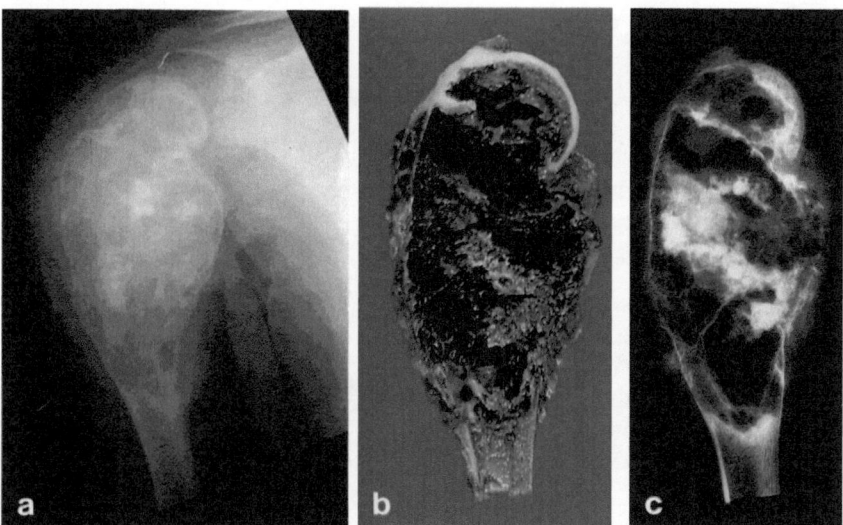

Fig. 25 a–c. *Telangiectatic osteosarcoma.* Female, 6 years. Upper third of humerus. **a** Radiograph. **b** Photograph of specimen. **c** Radiograph of specimen

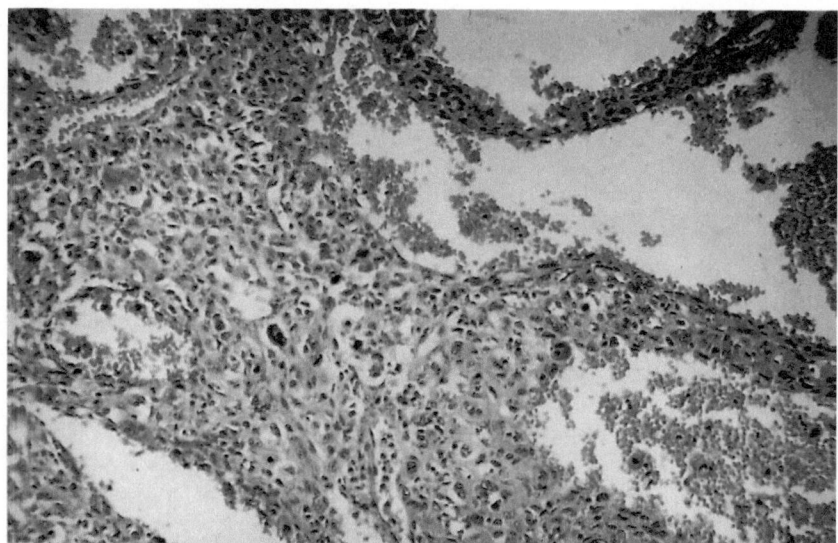

Fig. 26. *Telangiectatic osteosarcoma.* Same case as Fig. 25. Large blood-filled spaces

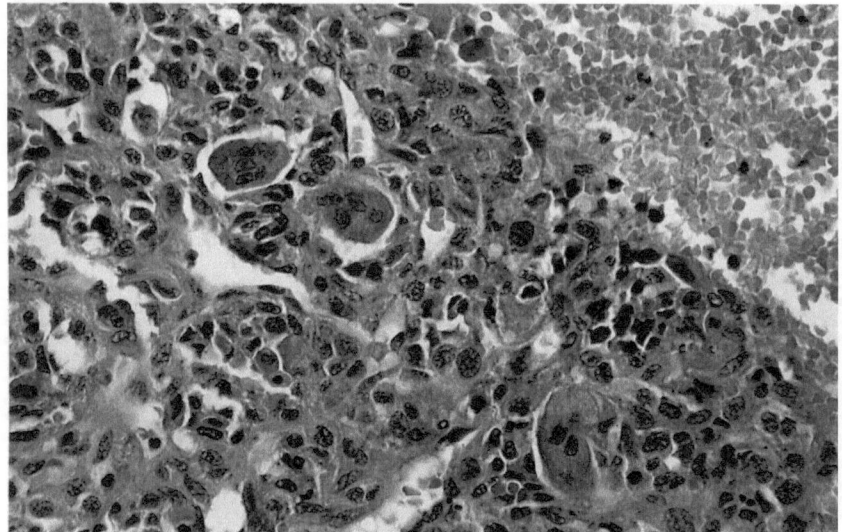

Fig. 27. *Telangiectatic osteosarcoma.* Same case as Fig. 25

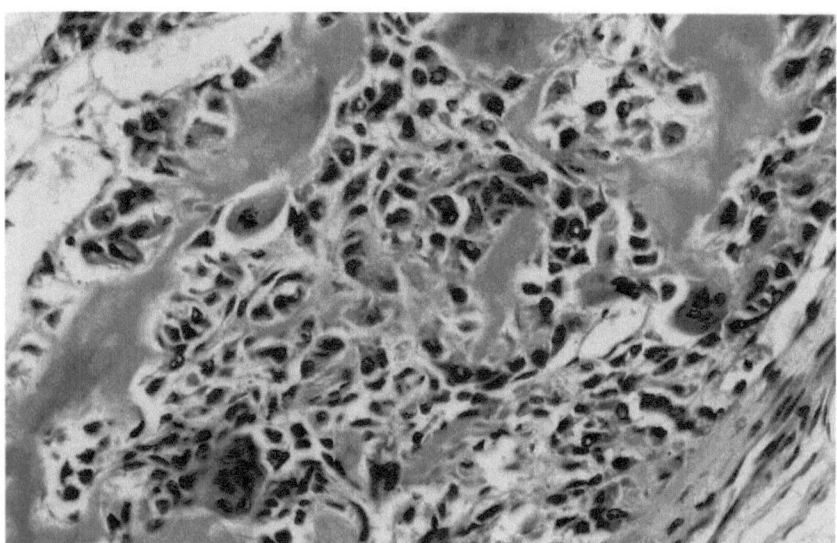

Fig. 28. *Telangiectatic osteosarcoma.* Same case as Fig. 25. Osteoid formed by tumour cells

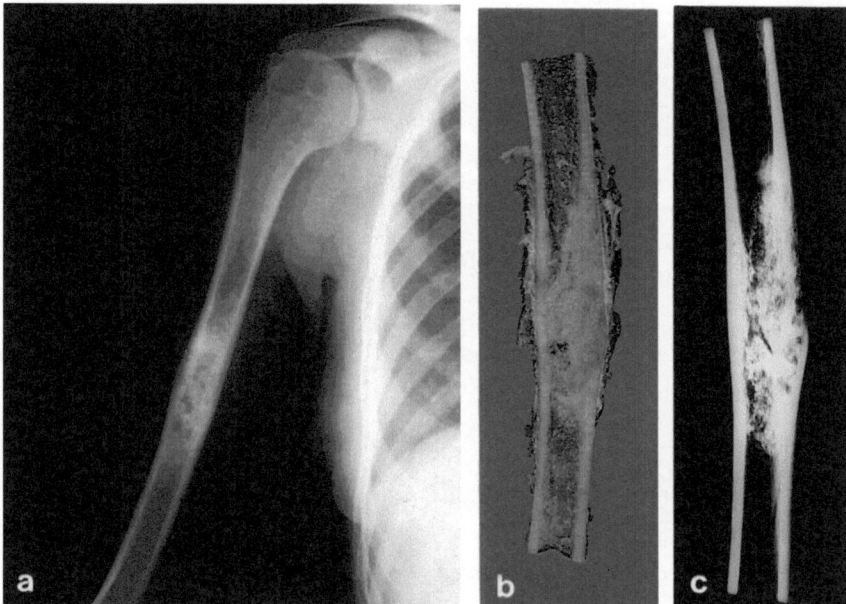

Fig. 29 a–c. *Intraosseous well-differentiated osteosarcoma.* Female, 15 years. Shaft of humerus. **a** Radiograph. **b** Photograph of specimen. **c** Radiograph of specimen

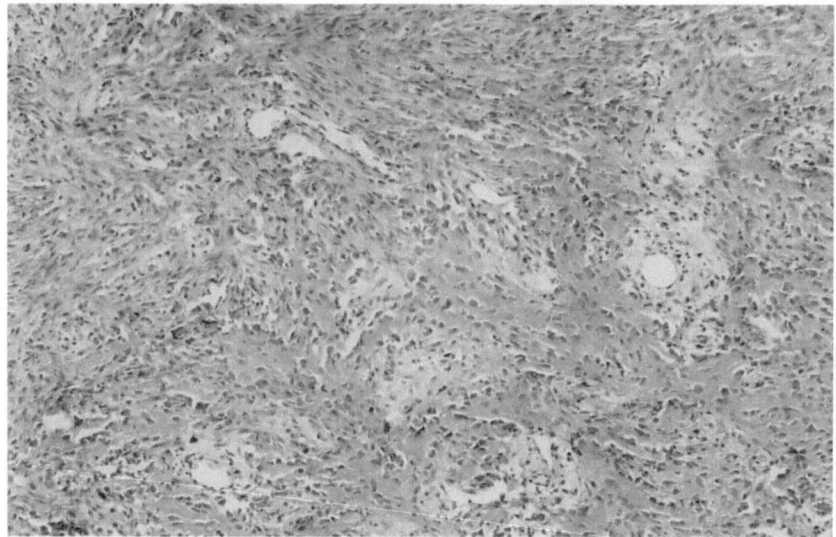

Fig. 30. *Intraosseous well-differentiated osteosarcoma.* Same case as Fig. 29. Simulates fibrous dysplasia at low power

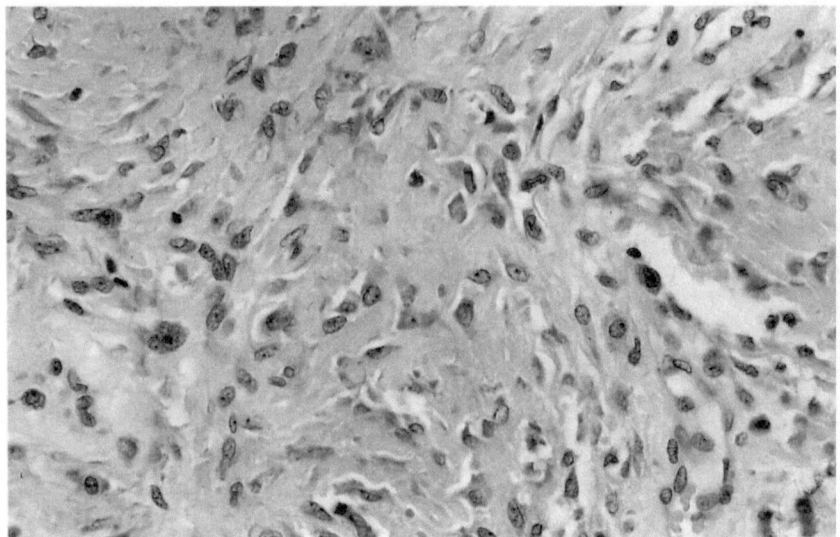

Fig. 31. *Intraosseous well-differentiated osteosarcoma.* Same case as Fig. 29

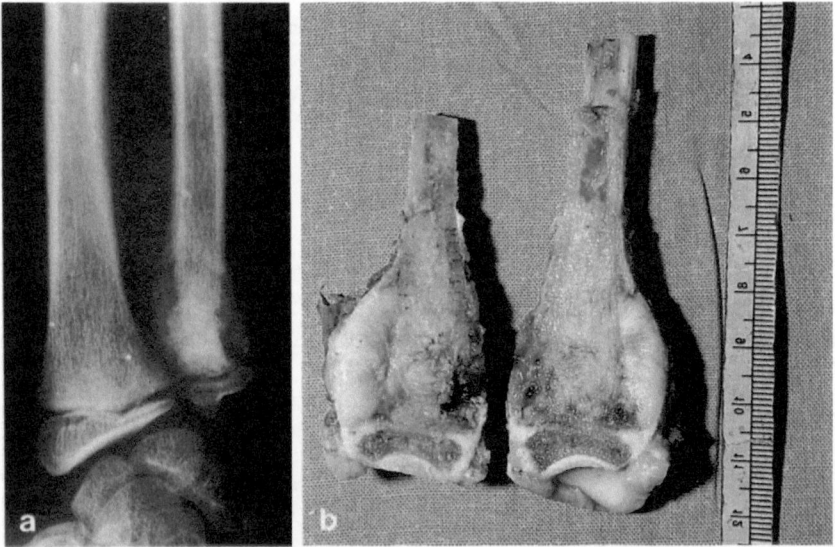

Fig. 32 a, b. *Round-cell osteosarcoma.* Male, 13 years. Distal end of ulna. **a** Radiograph. **b** Photograph of specimen

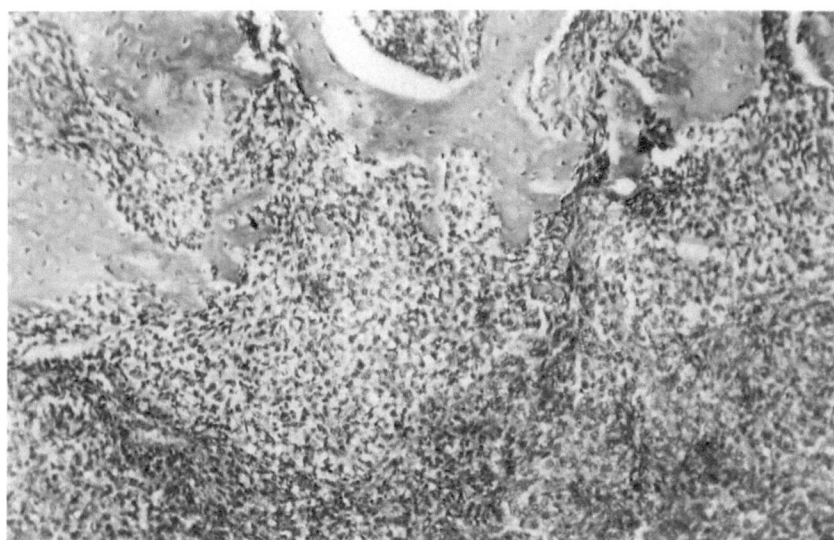

Fig. 33. *Round-cell osteosarcoma.* Same case as Fig. 32. Simulates Ewing sarcoma at low power

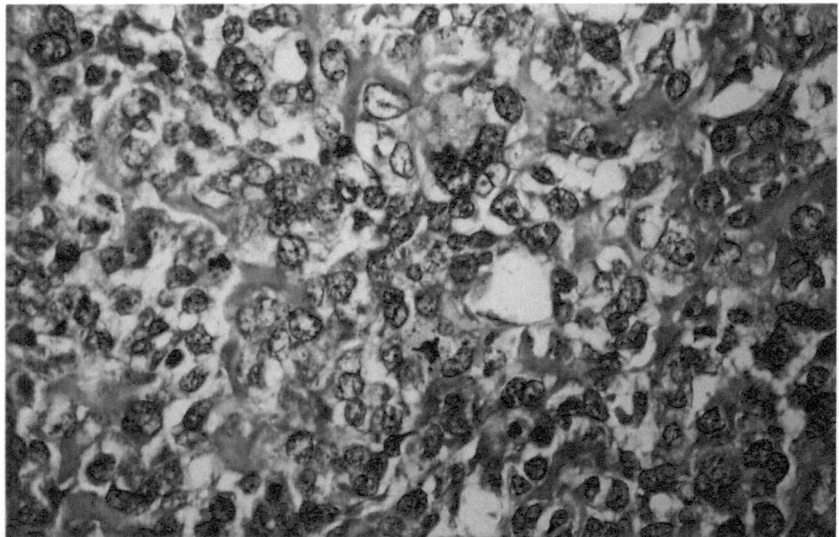

Fig. 34. *Round-cell osteosarcoma.* Same case as Fig. 32. Bone formed by round cells

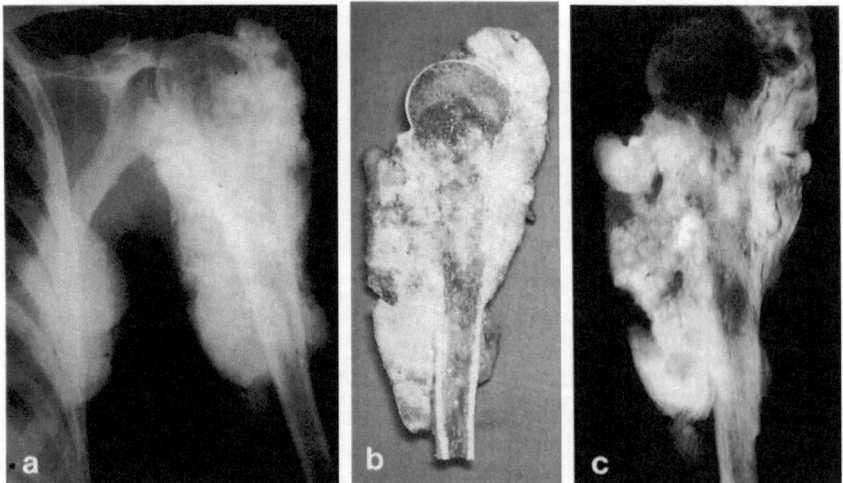

Fig. 35 a–c. *Parosteal osteosarcoma.* Female, 17 years. Upper shaft of humerus.
a Radiograph. **b** Photograph of specimen. **c** Radiograph of specimen

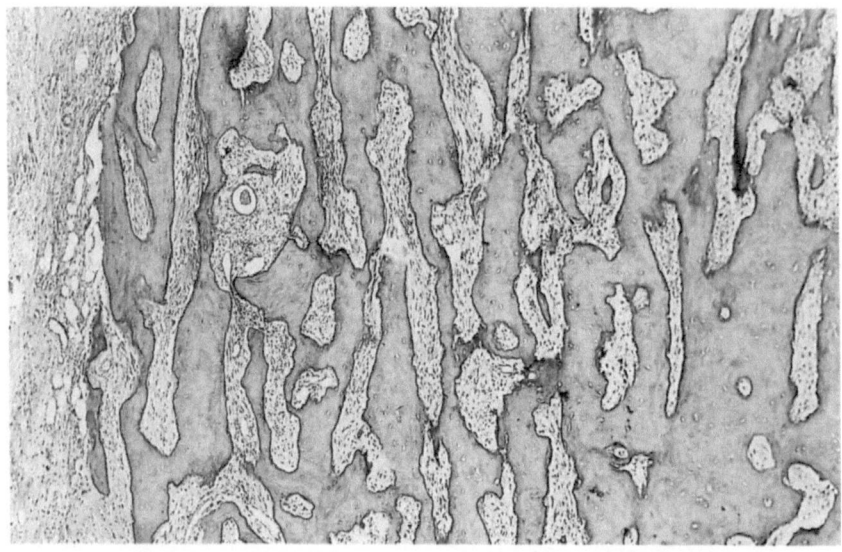

Fig. 36. *Parosteal osteosarcoma.* Same case as Fig. 35. Sclerotic bone of tumour

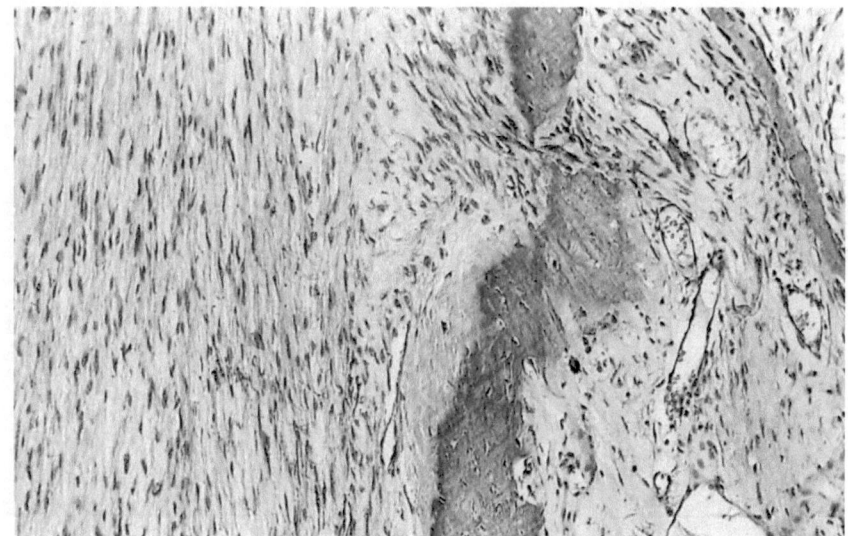

Fig. 37. *Parosteal osteosarcoma.* Same case as Fig. 35. Fibrosarcomatous tissue

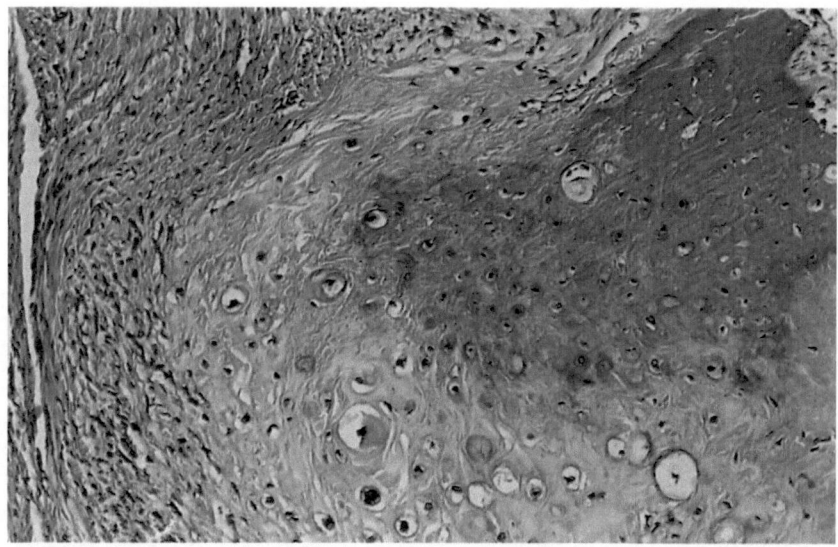

Fig. 38. *Parosteal osteosarcoma.* Same case as Fig. 35. Chondrosarcomatous tissue

62

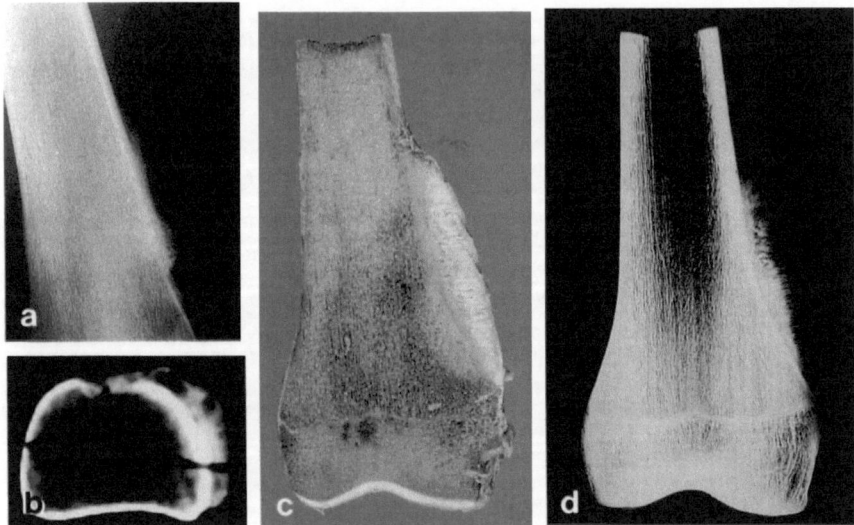

Fig. 39 a–d. *Periosteal osteosarcoma.* Male, 19 years. Lower metaphysis of femur. **a** Radiograph. **b** Tomogrram. **c** Photograph of specimen. **d** Radiograph
of specimen

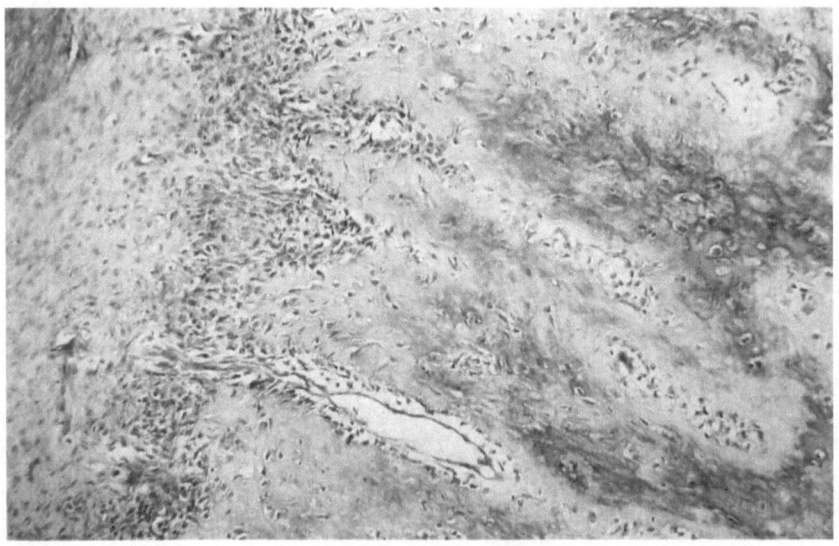

Fig. 40. *Periosteal osteosarcoma.* Same case as Fig. 39

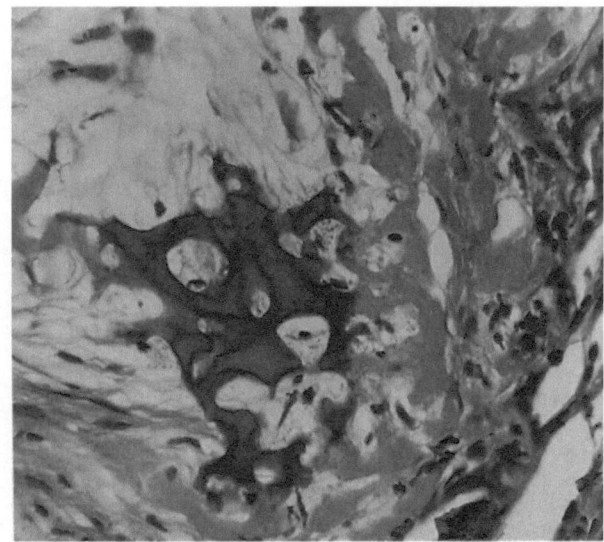

Fig. 41. *Periosteal osteosarcoma.* Same case as Fig. 39. Lace-like femoral bone

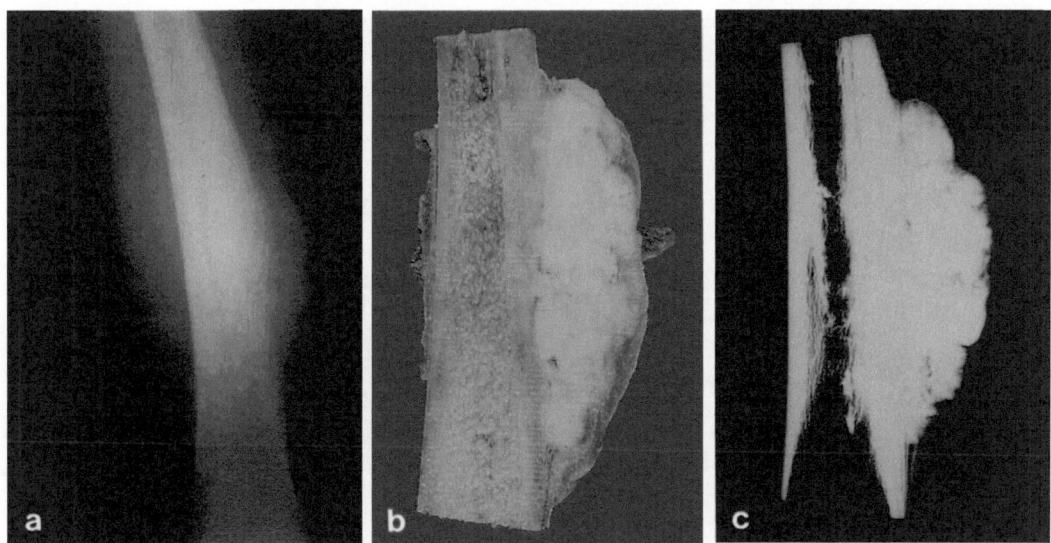

Fig. 42 a–c. *High-grade surface osteosarcoma.* Female, 13 years. Shaft of femur.
a Radiograph. **b** Photograph of specimen. **c** Radiograph of specimen

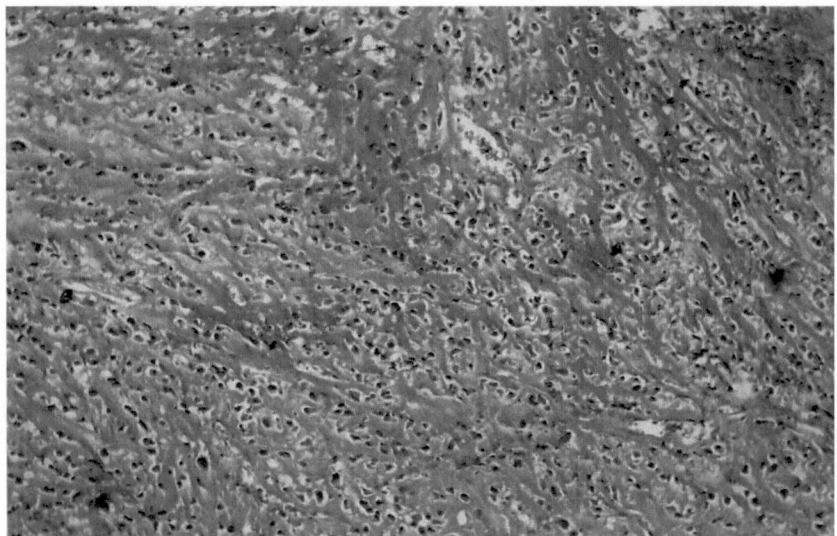

Fig. 43. *High-grade surface osteosarcoma.* Same case as Fig. 42

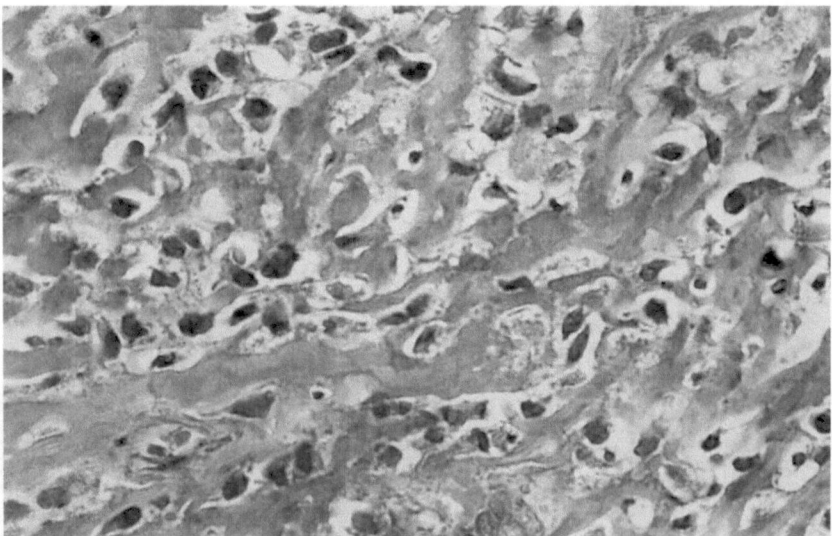

Fig. 44. *High-grade surface osteosarcoma.* Same case as Fig. 42. Highly pleomorphic area

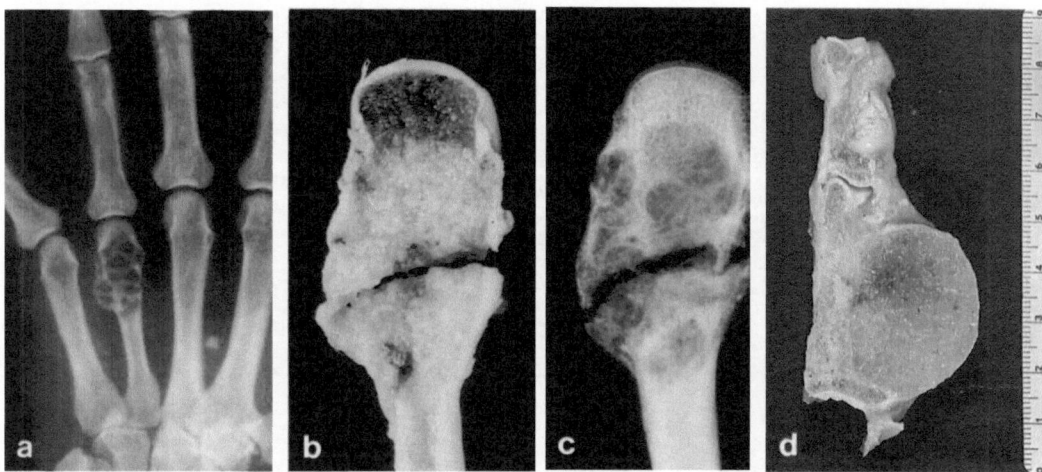

Fig. 45 a–d. *Enchondroma.* **a–c** Male, 64 years. Metacarpal. **a** Radiograph. **b** Photograph of specimen. **c** Radiograph of specimen. **d** Photograph of another specimen

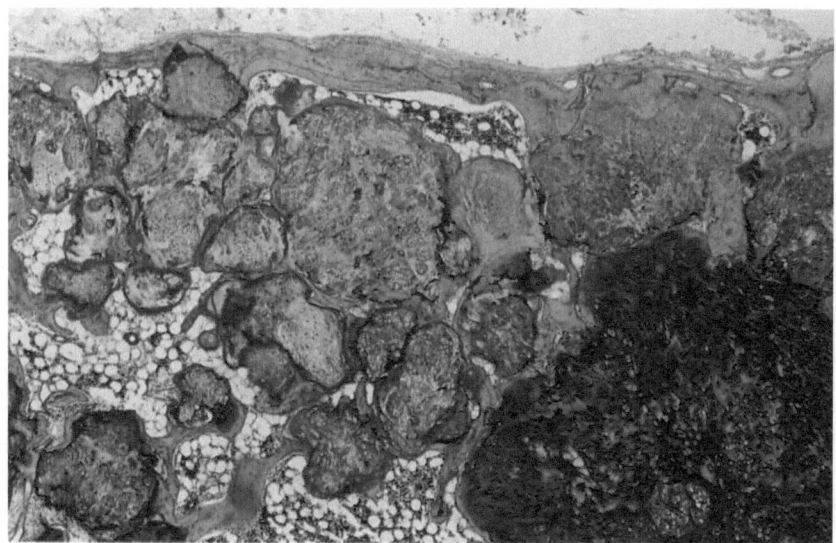

Fig. 46. *Chondroma.* Same case as Fig. 45 a–c

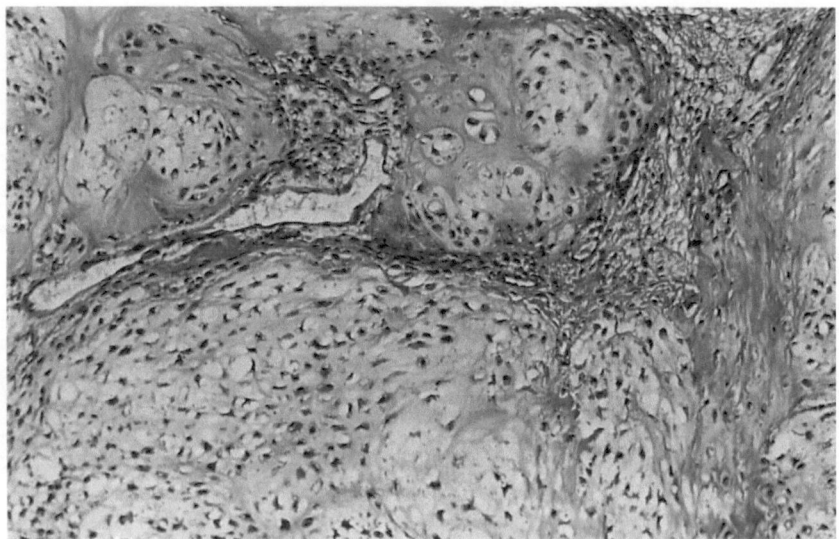

Fig. 47. *Chondroma.* Same case as Fig. 45 a–c

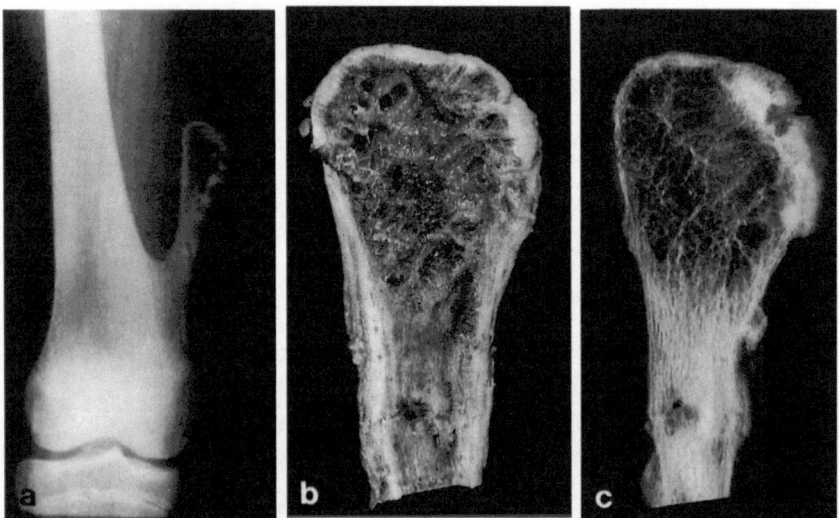

Fig. 48 a–c. *Osteochondroma.* Female, 10 years. Lower metaphysis of femur.
a Radiograph. **b** Photograph of specimen. **c** Radiograph of specimen

67

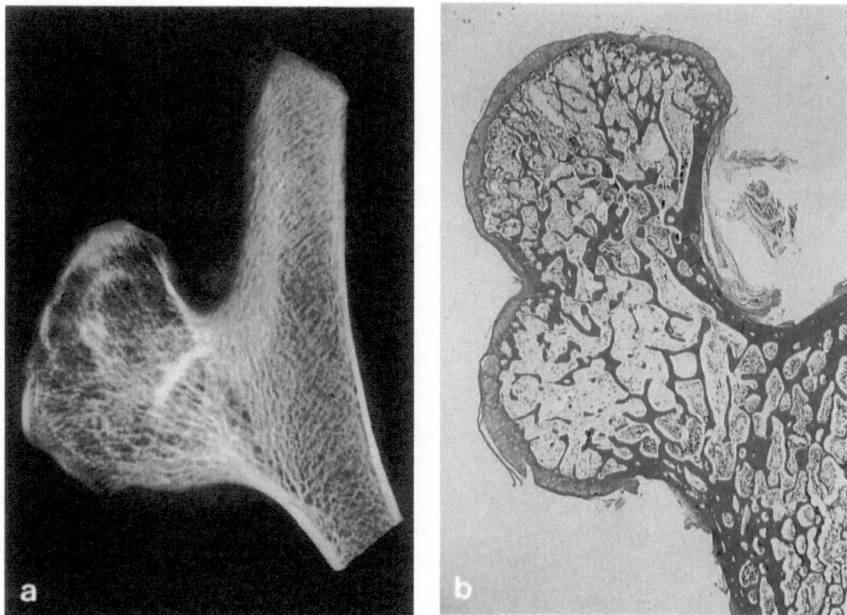

Fig. 49 a, b. *Osteochondroma.* Male, 13 years. Ilium. **a** Radiograph of specimen.
b Same case as **a**

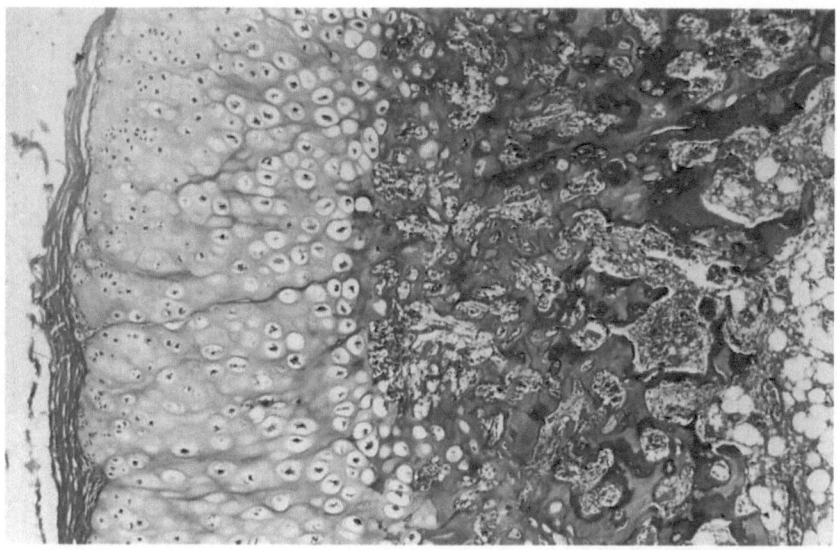

Fig. 50. *Osteochondroma.* Same case as Fig. 49

68

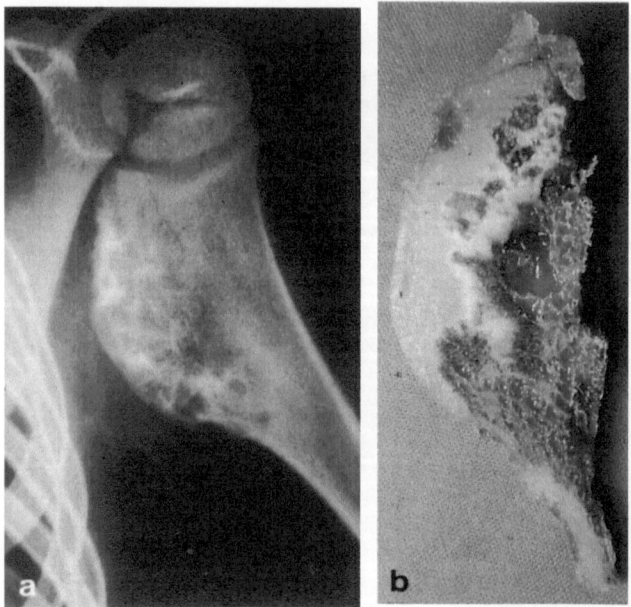

Fig. 51 a, b. *Osteochondroma.* Male, 6 years. Upper metaphysis of humerus. **a** Radiograph. **b** Photograph of specimen

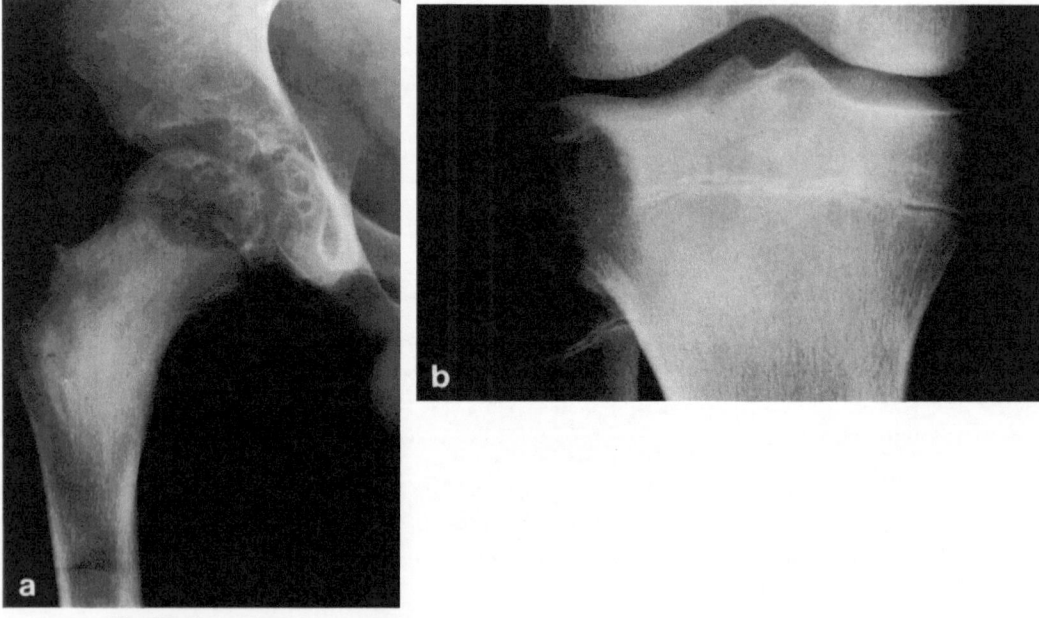

Fig. 52 a, b. *Chondroblastoma.* **a** Male, 11 years. Upper epiphysis of femur. Radiograph. **b** Male, 14 years. Upper epiphysis of tibia. Radiograph

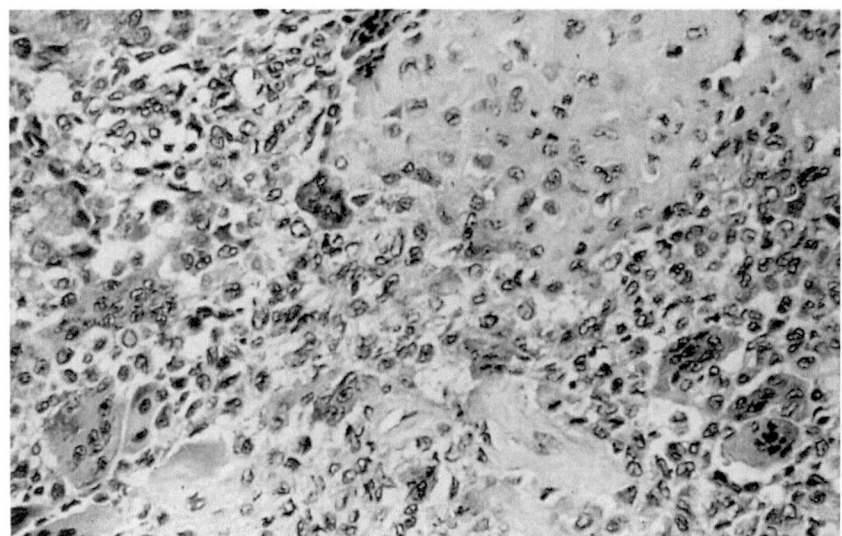

Fig. 53. *Chondroblastoma.* Same case as Fig. 52 b

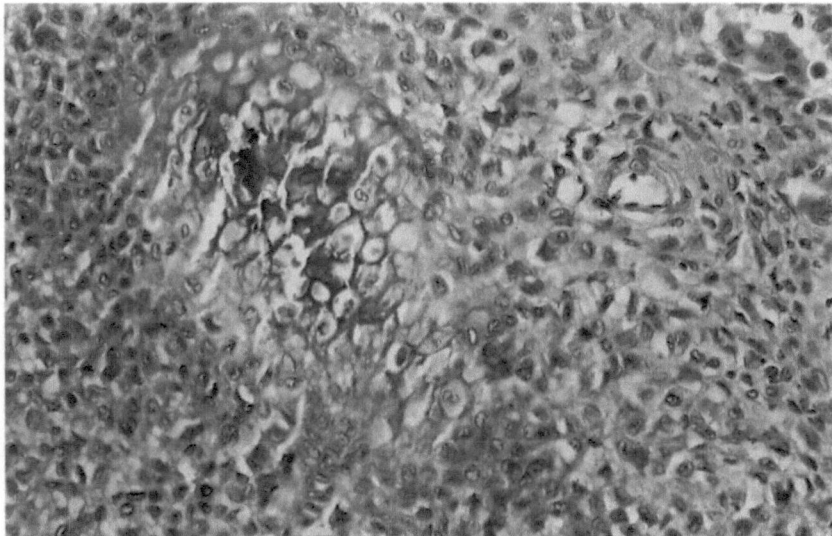

Fig. 54. *Chondroblastoma.* Same case as Fig. 52 b

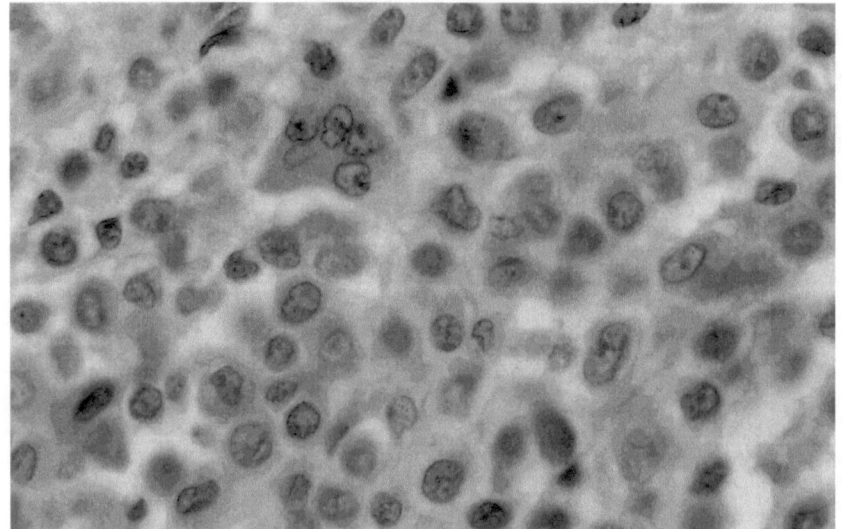

Fig. 55. *Chondroblastoma.* Same case as Fig. 52 b

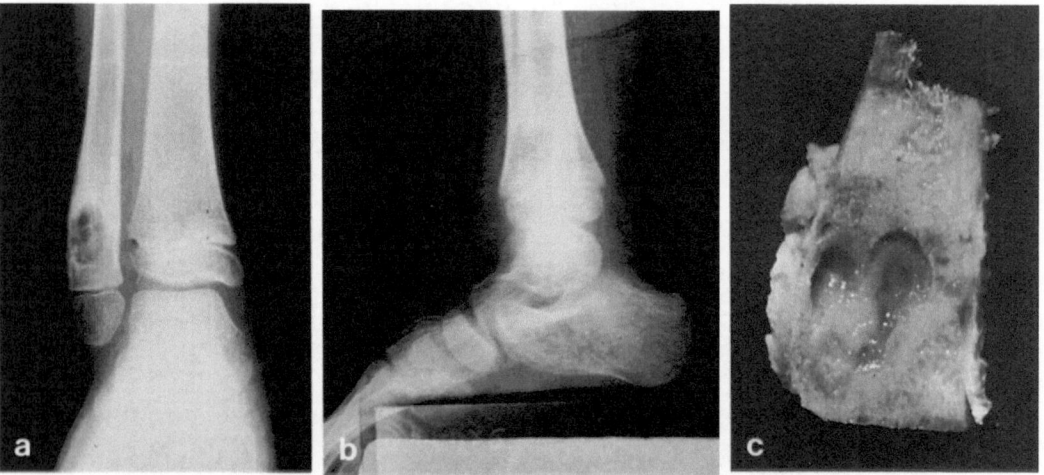

Fig. 56 a–c. *Chondromyxoid fibroma.* Male, 9 years. Lower metaphysis of fibula.
a, b Radiographs. **c** Photograph of specimen

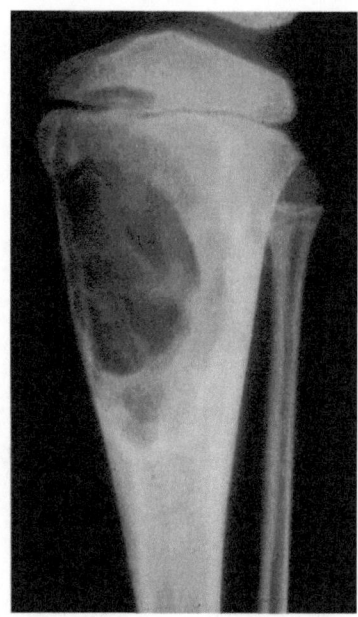

Fig.57. *Chondromyxoid fibroma.* Male, 10 years. Upper metaphysis of tibia. Radiograph

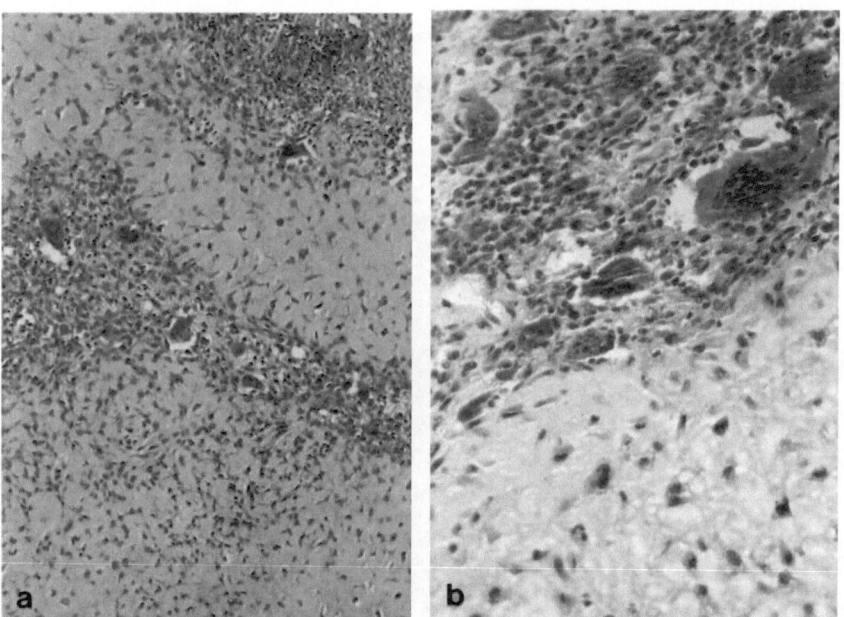

Fig.58 a,b. *Chondromyxoid fibroma.* Same case as Fig.57. Chondroid stroma

72

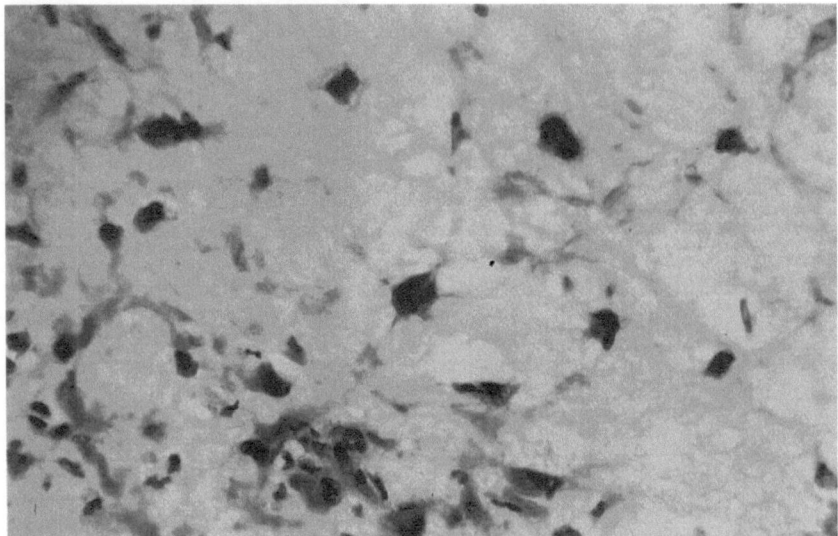

Fig. 59. *Chondromyxoid fibroma.* Same case as Fig. 57. Myxoid stroma

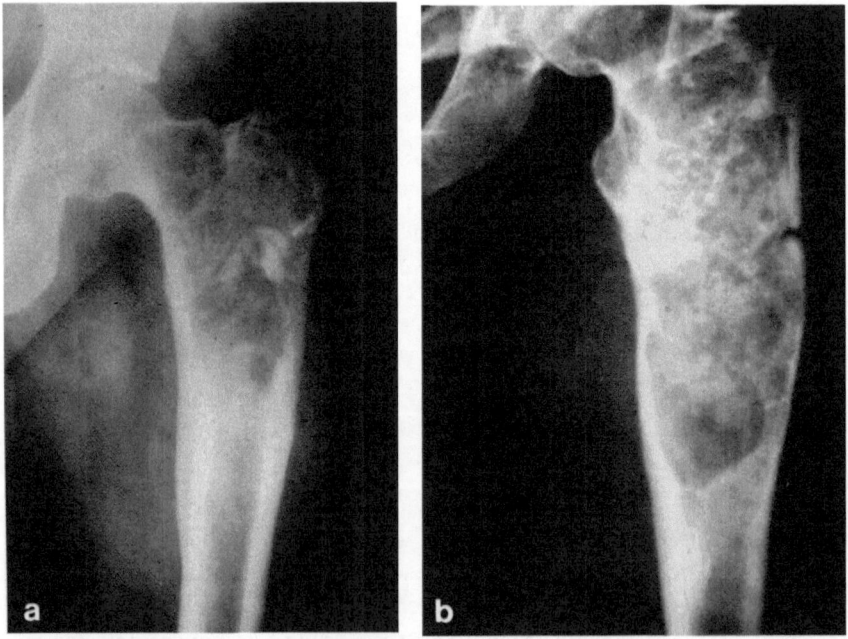

Fig. 60 a, b. *Chondrosarcoma.* **a** Male, 28 years. Upper shaft of femur. Radiograph. **b** Male, 38 years. Upper shaft of femur. Radiograph

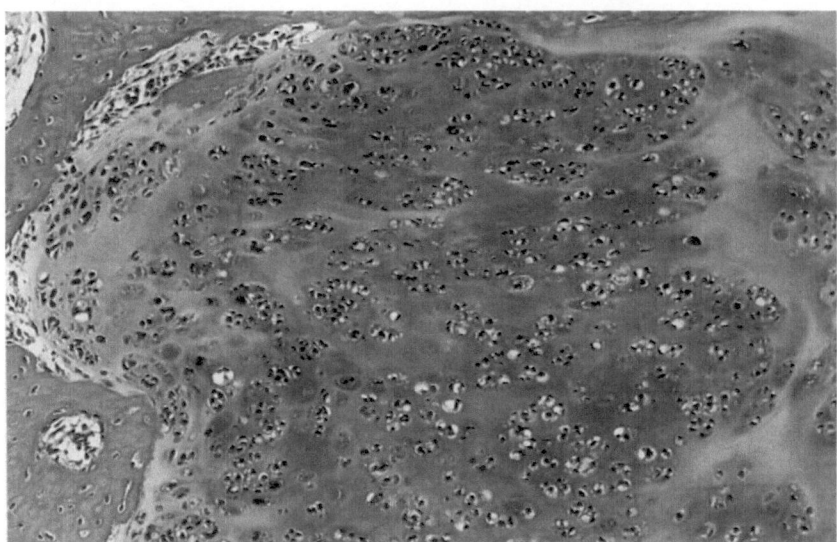

Fig. 61. *Chondrosarcoma.* Well-differentiated tumour

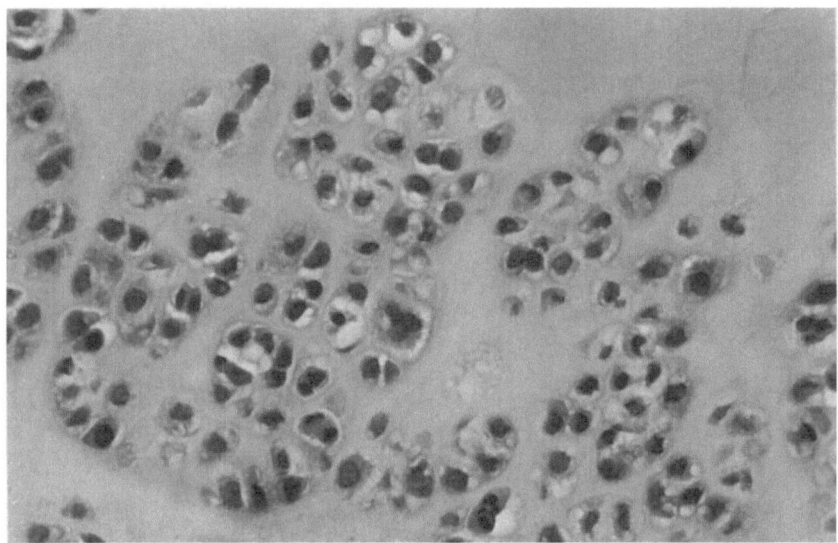

Fig. 62. *Chondrosarcoma.* Same case as Fig. 61

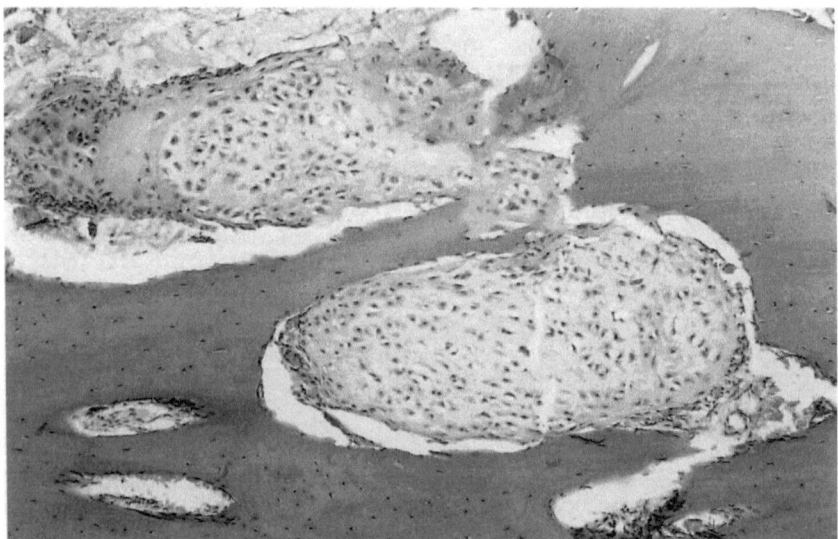

Fig. 63. *Chondrosarcoma.* Cortical erosion

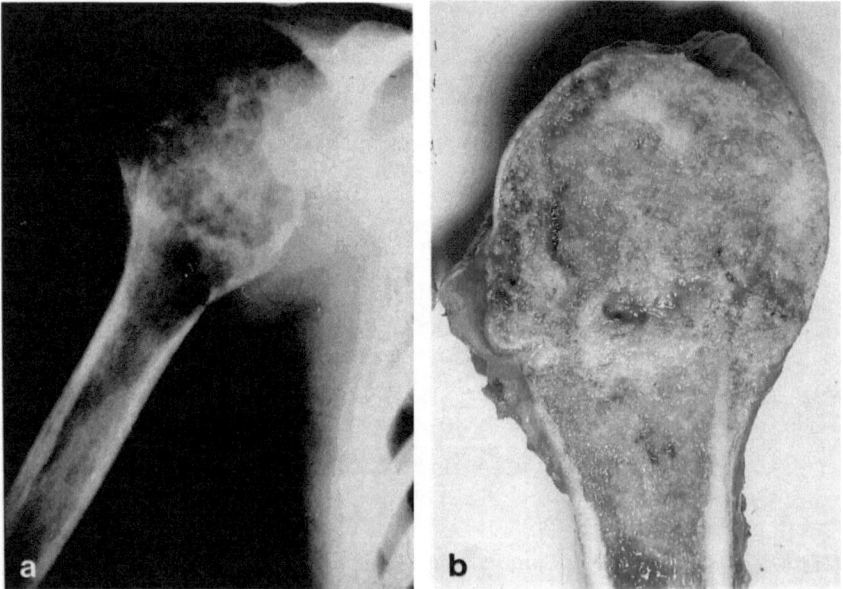

Fig. 64 a, b. *Chondrosarcoma.* Female, 24 years. Upper end of humerus. **a** Radiograph. **b** Photograph of specimen

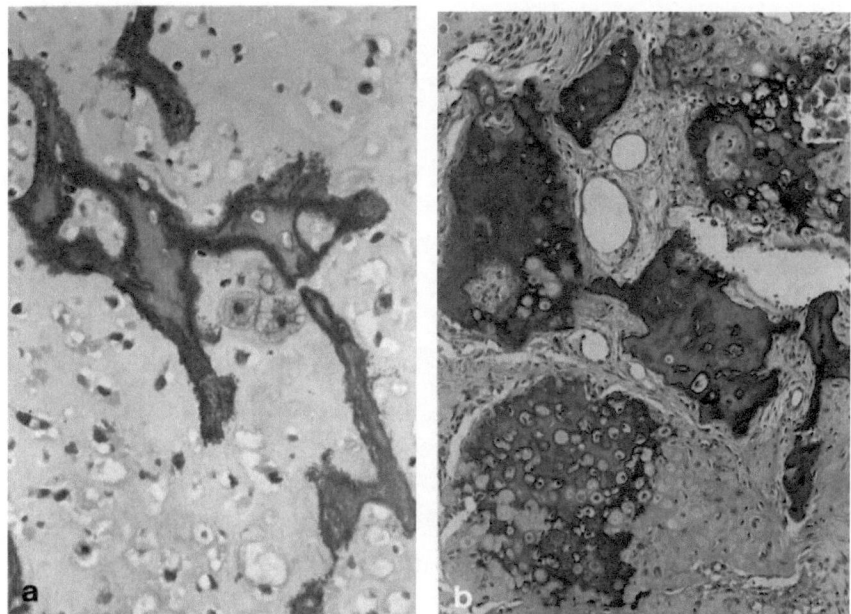

Fig. 65 a, b. *Chondrosarcoma.* **a** Metaplastic ossification. **b** Calcification and endochondral ossification

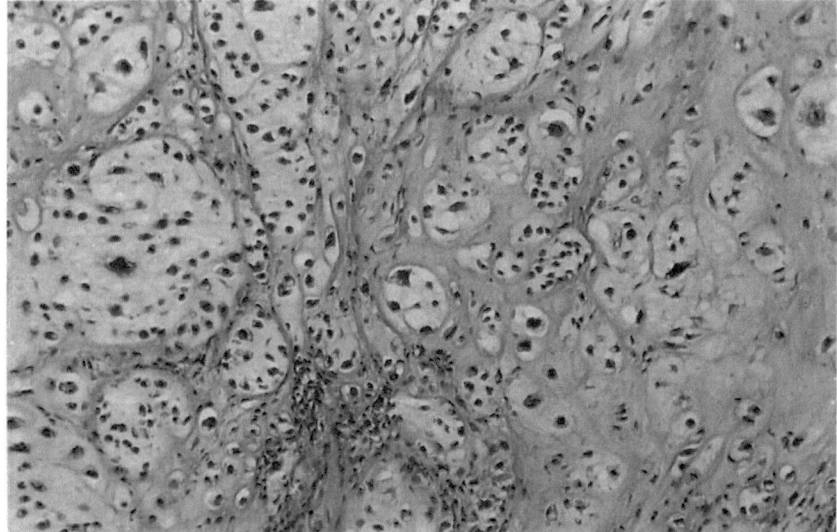

Fig. 66. *Chondrosarcoma.* Pleomorphic cartilage

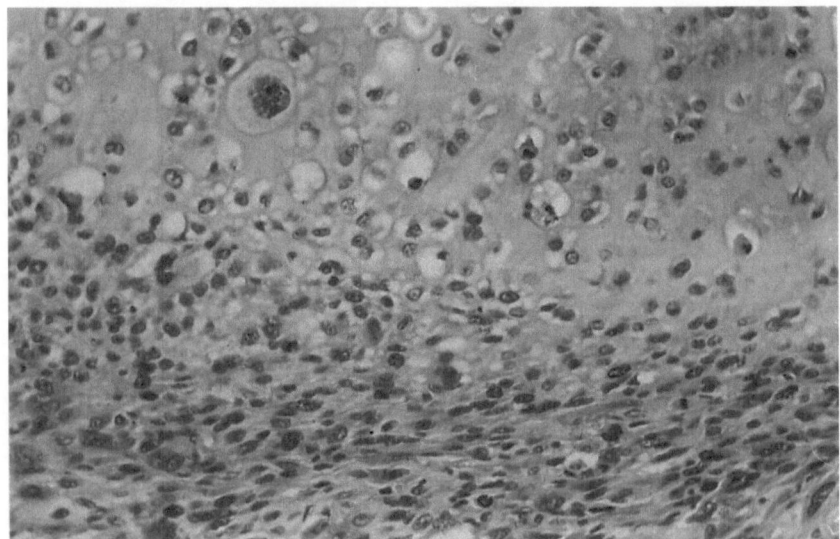

Fig. 67. *Chondrosarcoma.* Spindle-cell pattern

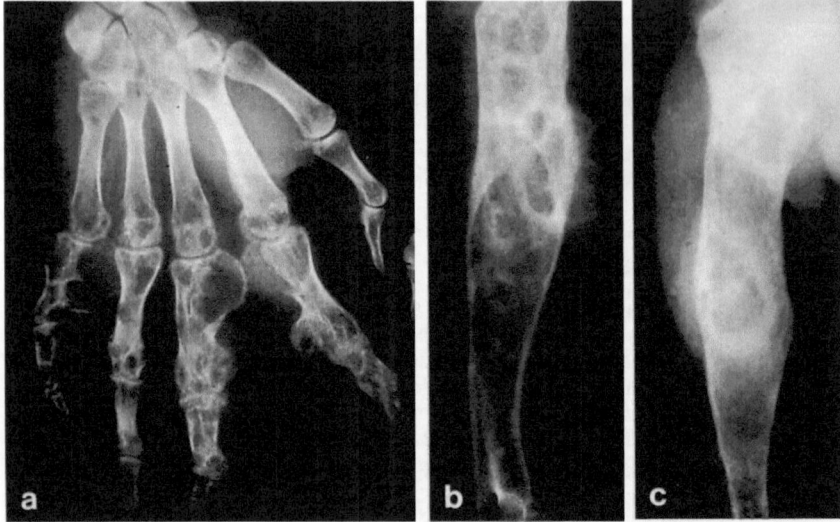

Fig. 68 a–c. *Chondrosarcoma in Ollier disease.* Male, 21 years. **a** Hand with multiple enchondromas. Radiograph. **b, c** Humerus with chondrosarcoma. Radiographs

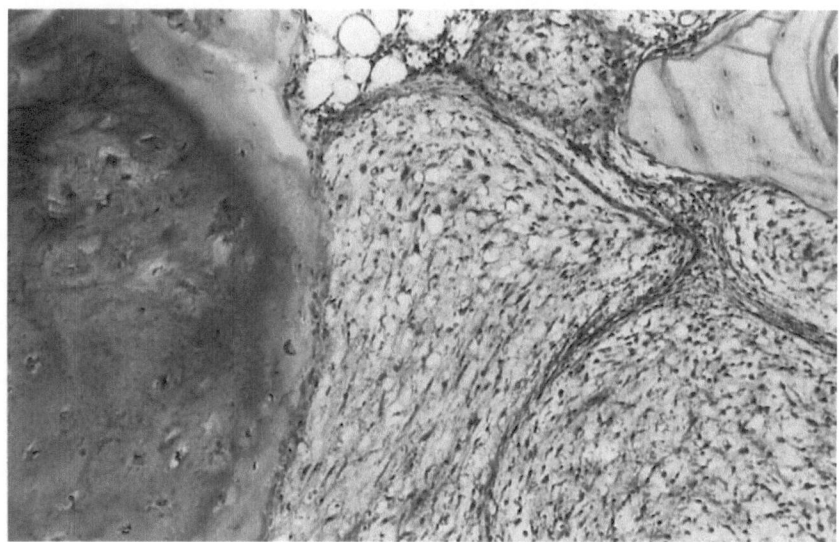

Fig. 69. *Chondrosarcoma in Ollier disease.* Same case as Fig. 68 b, c. Field showing enchondroma and chondrosarcoma

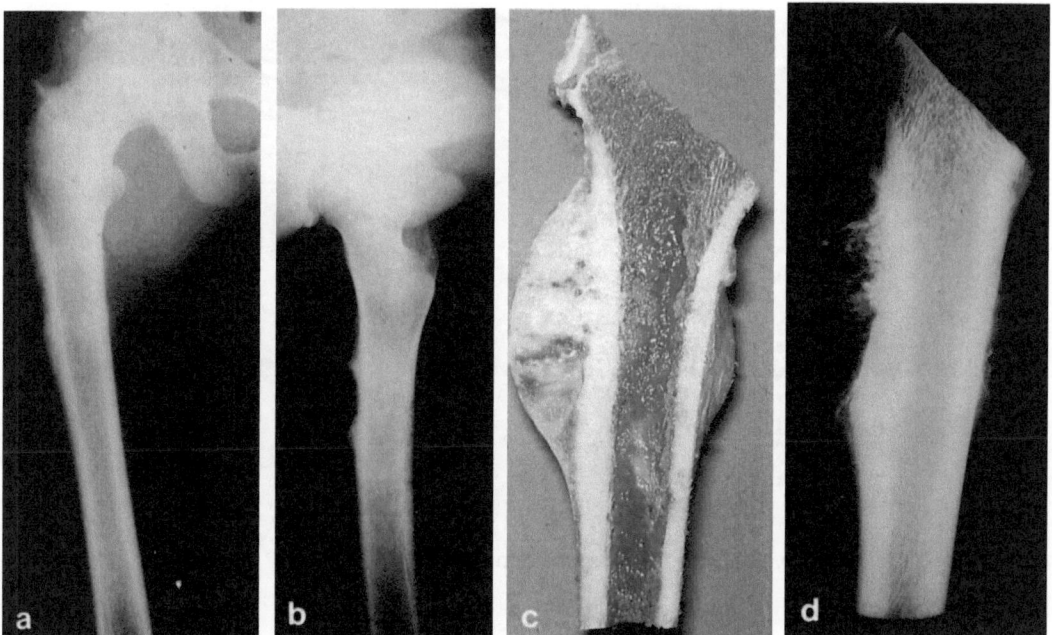

Fig. 70 a–d. *Juxtacortical chondrosarcoma.* Male, 17 years. Upper shaft of femur.
a, b Radiographs. **c** Photograph of specimen. **d** Radiograph of specimen

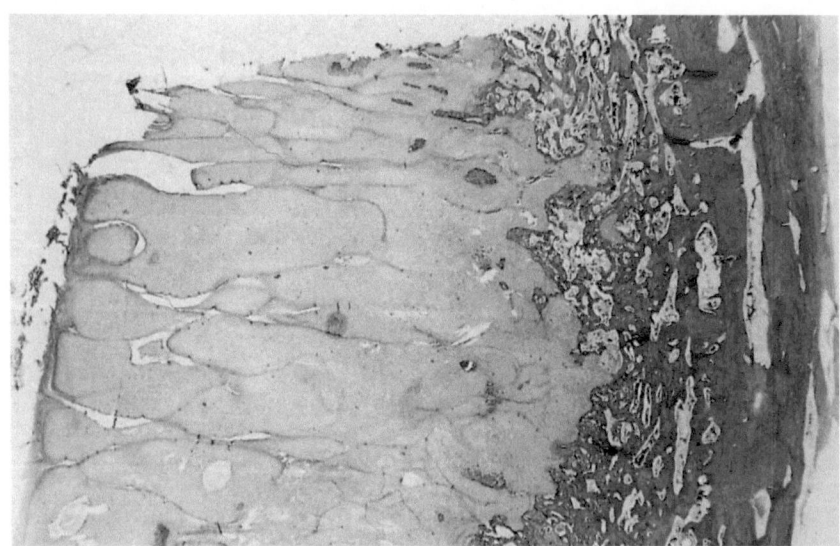

Fig. 71. *Juxtacortical chondrosarcoma.* Same case as Fig. 70

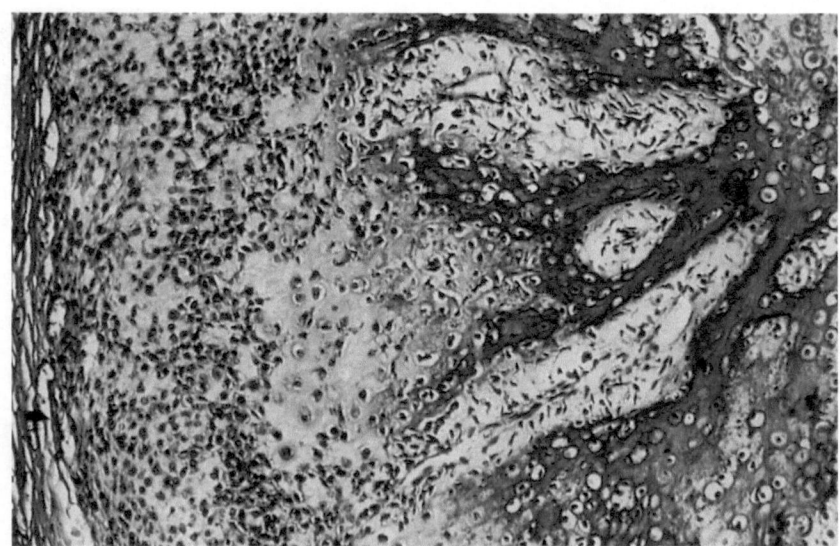

Fig. 72. *Juxtacortical chondrosarcoma.* Same case as Fig. 70

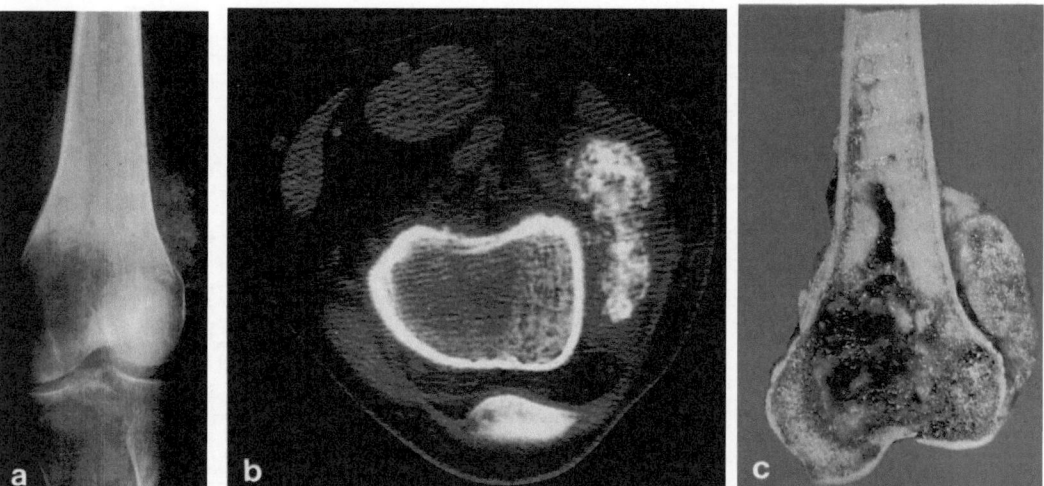

Fig. 73 a–c. *Mesenchymal chondrosarcoma.* Male, 36 years. Distal end of femur.
a Radiograph. **b** Tomogram. **c** Photograph of specimen

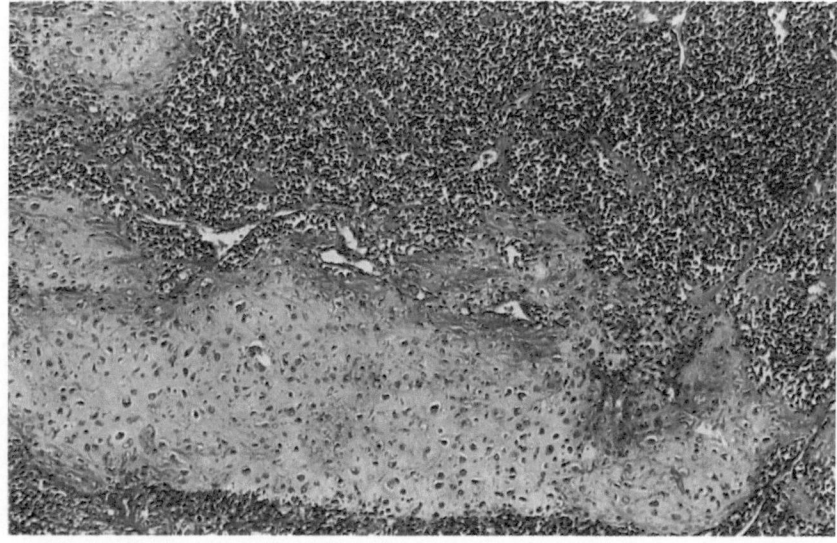

Fig. 74. *Mesenchymal chondrosarcoma.* Same case as Fig. 73

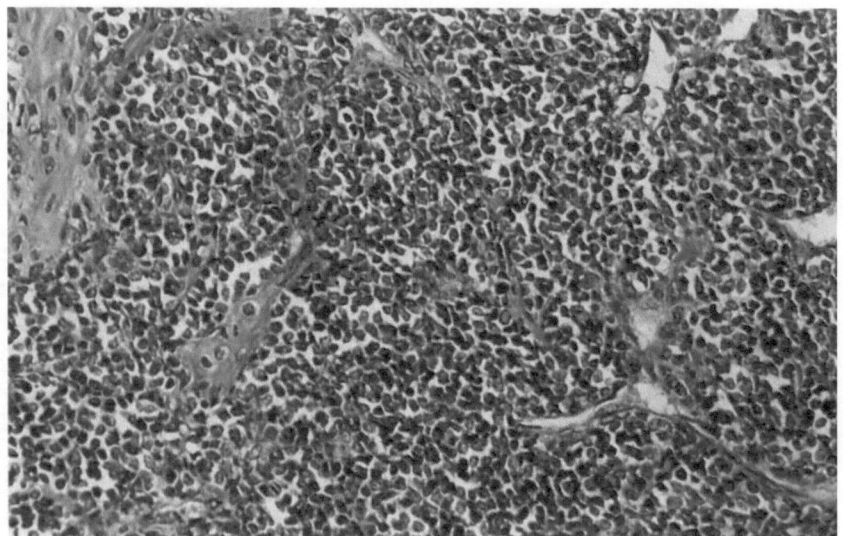

Fig. 75. *Mesenchymal chondrosarcoma.* Same case as Fig. 73. Poorly differentiated cells

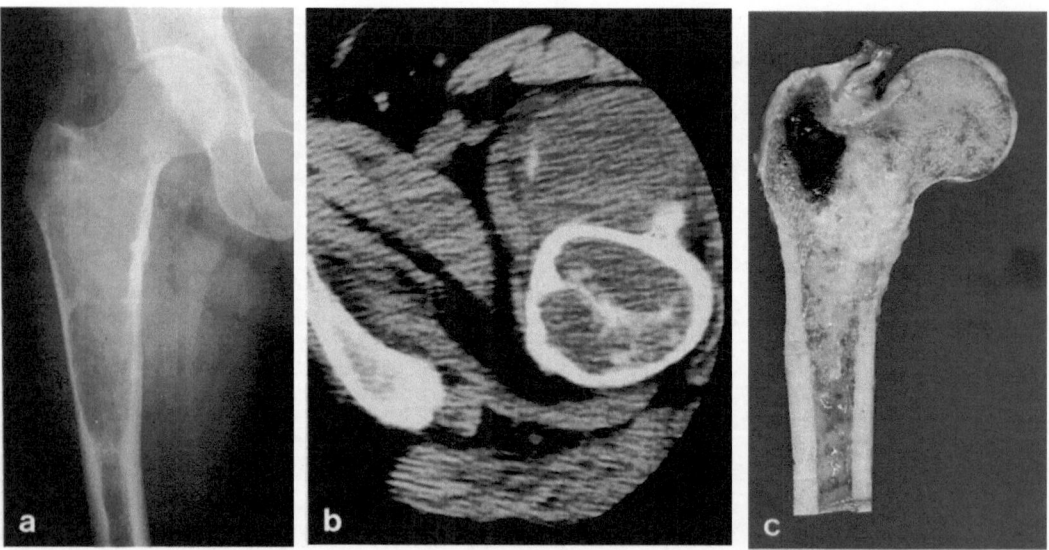

Fig. 76 a–c. *Dedifferentiated chondrosarcoma.* Male, 49 years. Upper shaft of femur. **a** Radiograph. **b** Tomogram. **c** Photograph of specimen

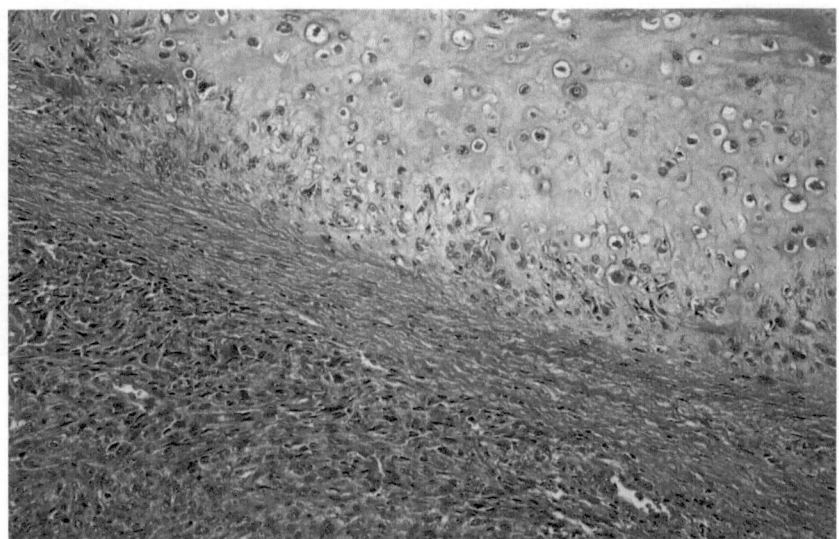

Fig. 77. *Dedifferentiated chondrosarcoma.* Same case as Fig. 76. Abrupt transition between low-grade cartilage tumour and dedifferentiated cells

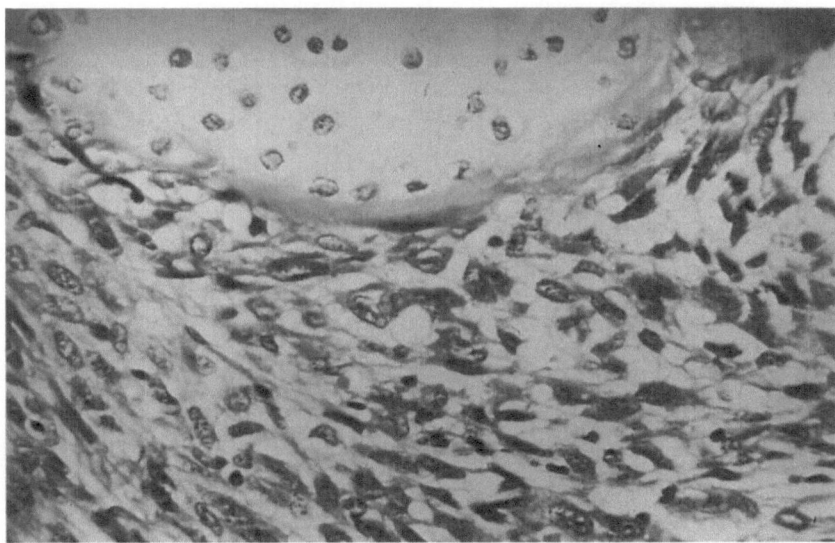

Fig. 78. *Dedifferentiated chondrosarcoma.* Same case as Fig. 76

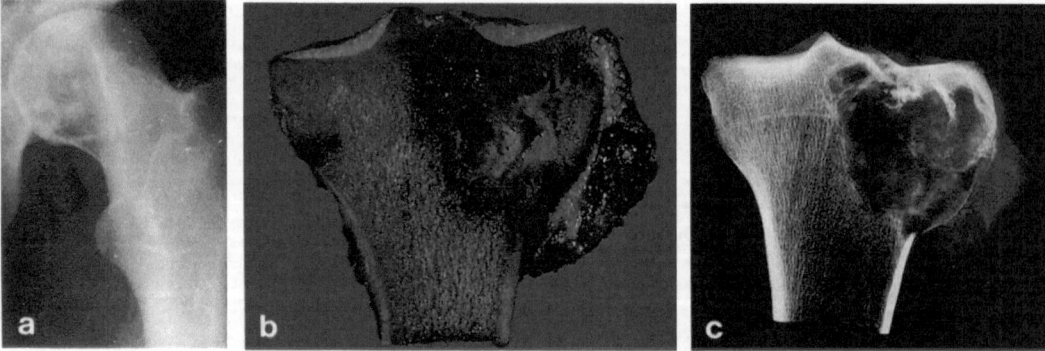

Fig. 79 a–c. *Clear-cell chondrosarcoma.* **a** Male, 76 years. Upper epiphysis of femur. Radiograph. **b,c** Male, 30 years. Upper end of tibia **b** Photograph of specimen. **c** Radiograph of specimen

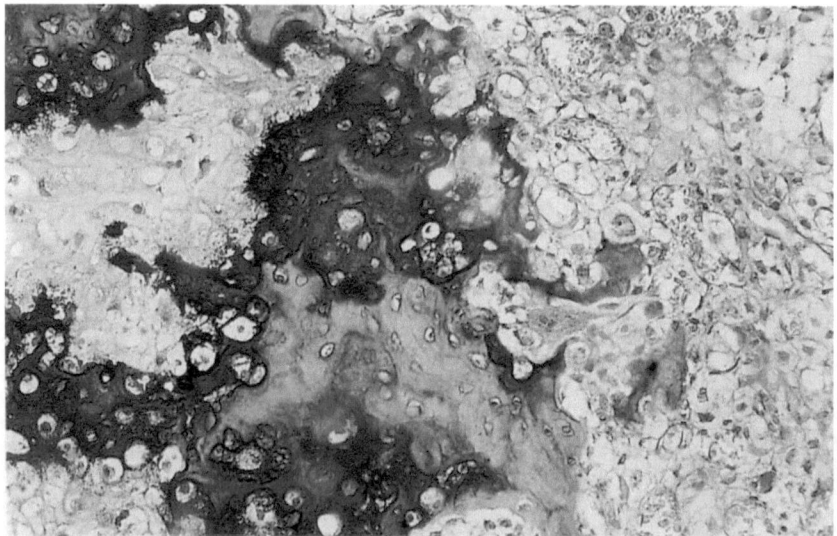

Fig. 80. *Clear-cell chondrosarcoma.* Same case as Fig. 79 b, c

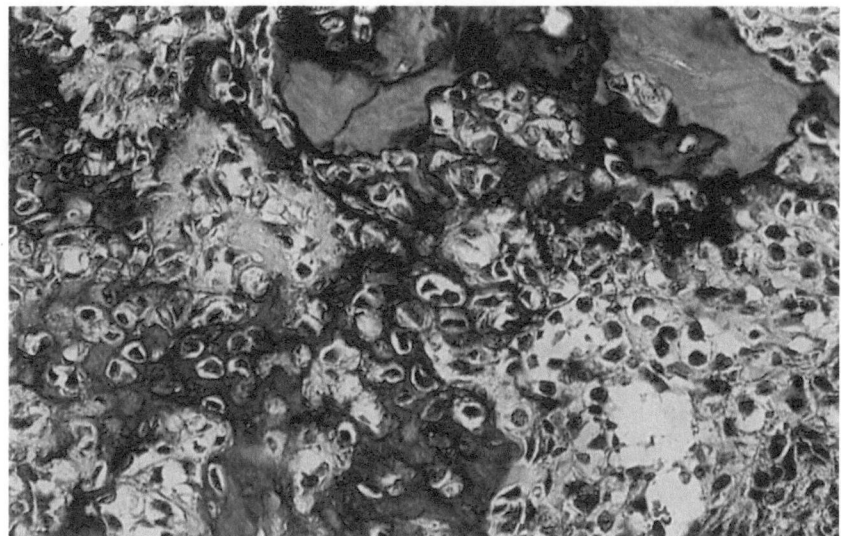

Fig. 81. *Clear-cell chondrosarcoma.* Same case as Fig. 79 b, c

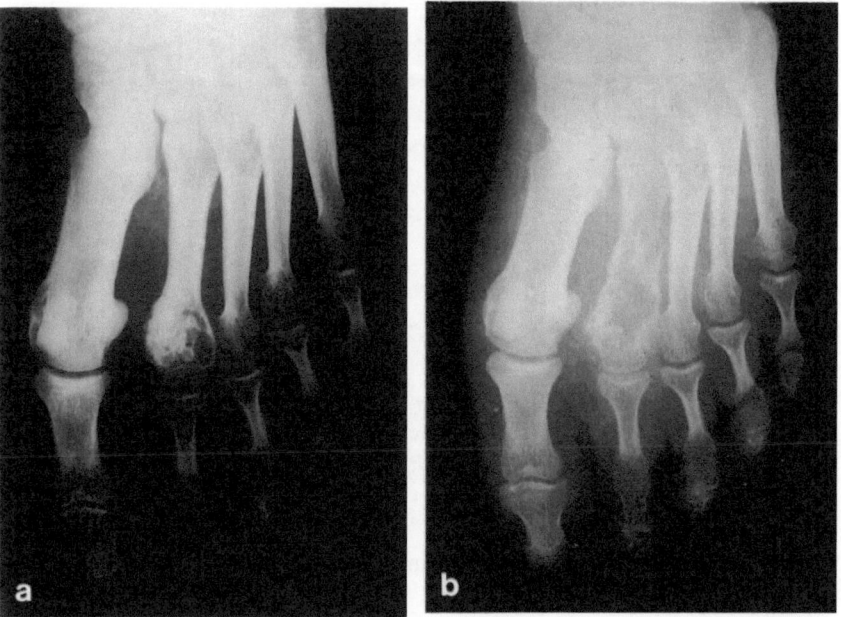

Fig. 82 a, b. *Malignant chondroblastoma?* Female, 32 years. Distal epiphysis of second metatarsal. **a** Radiograph. **b** Radiograph. Recurrence 5 months later

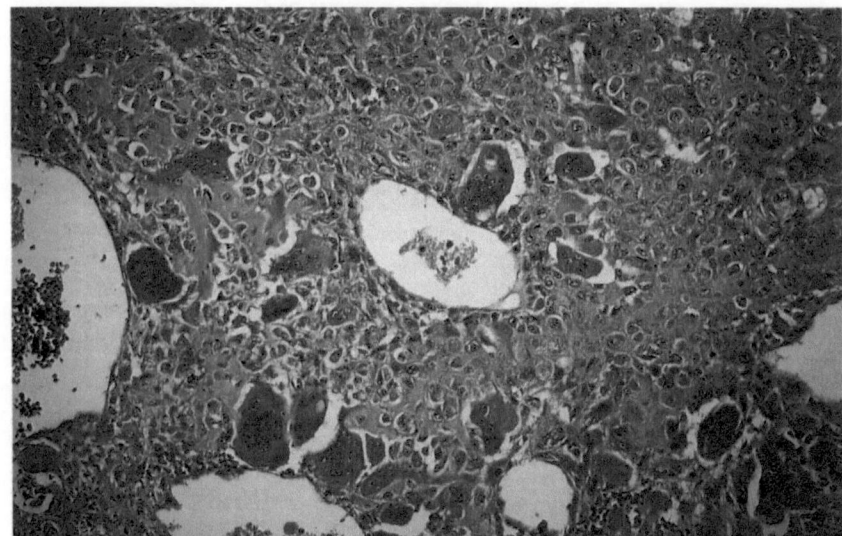

Fig. 83. *Malignant chondroblastoma?* Same case as Fig. 82 b

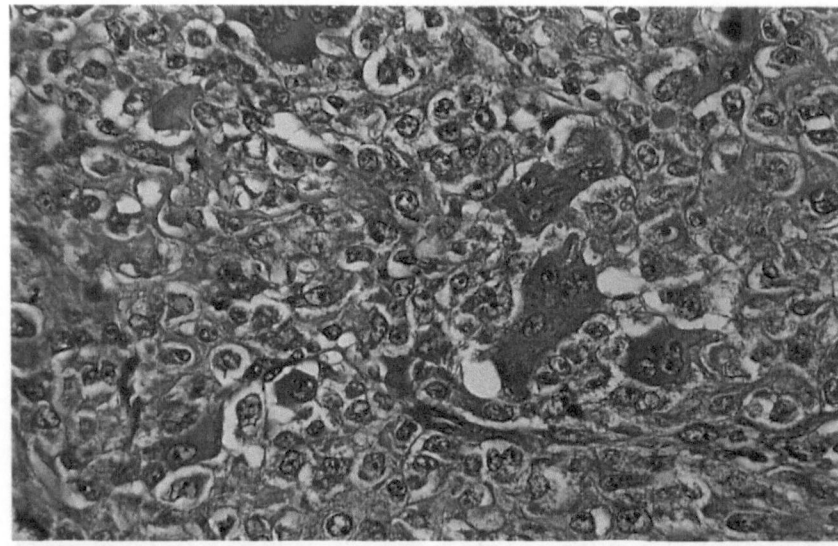

Fig. 84. *Malignant chondroblastoma?* Same case as Fig. 82 b. Giant cells between round cells are pleomorphic

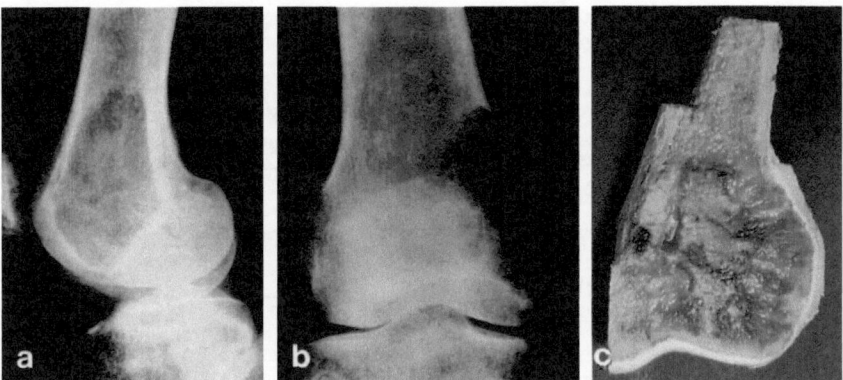

Fig. 85 a–c. *Giant-cell tumour.* Male, 56 years. Lower end of femur. **a,b** Radiographs. **c** Photograph of specimen

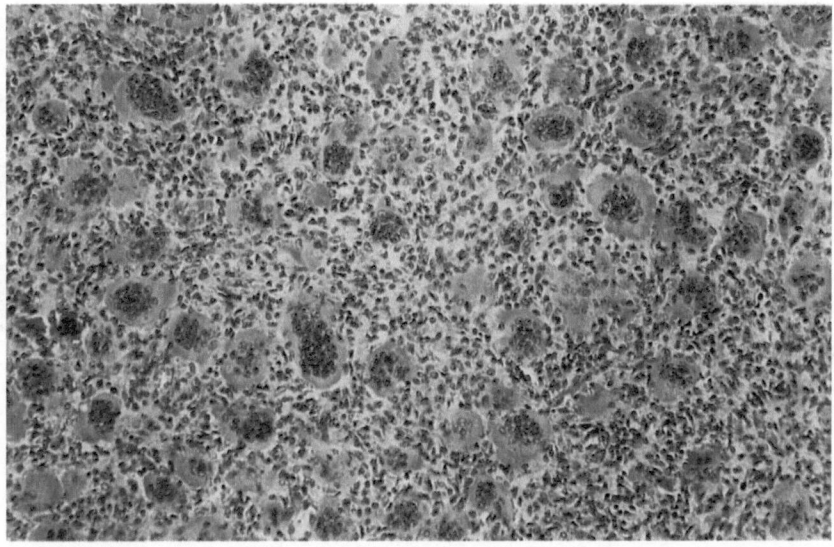

Fig. 86. *Giant-cell tumour.* Same case as Fig. 85

86

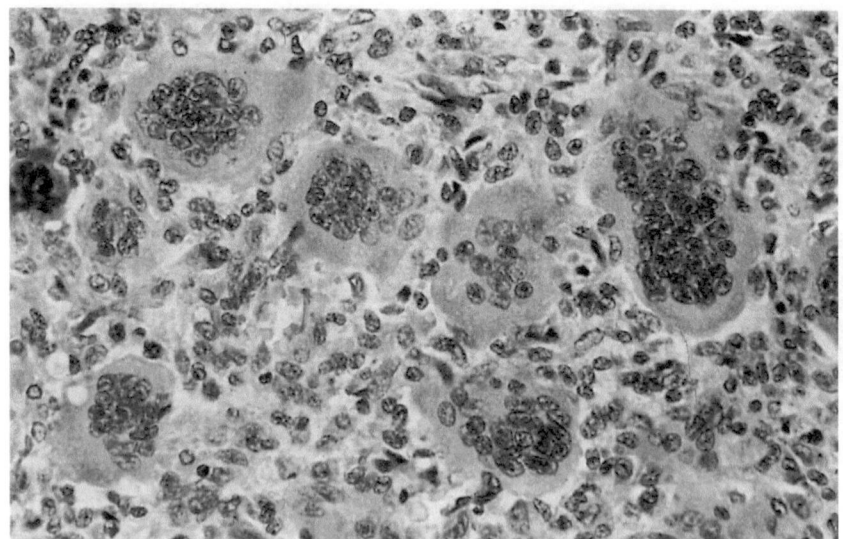

Fig. 87. *Giant-cell tumour.* Same case as Fig. 85

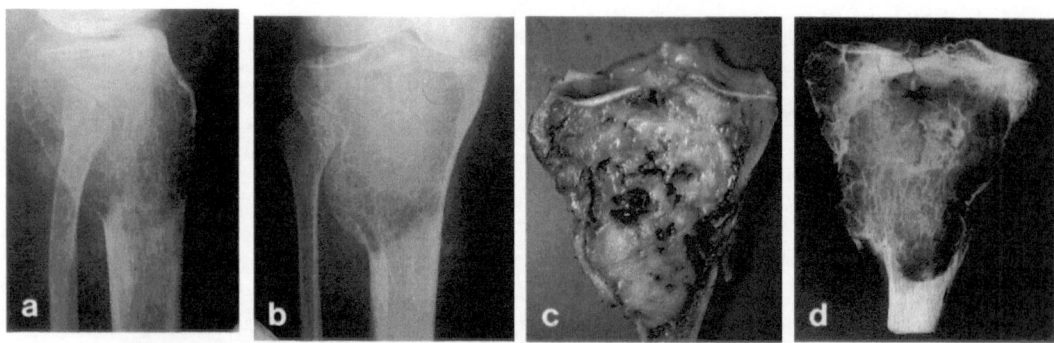

Fig. 88 a–d. *Giant-cell tumour.* Female, 30 years. Upper end of tibia. **a,b** Radiographs. **c** Photograph of specimen. **d** Radiograph of specimen

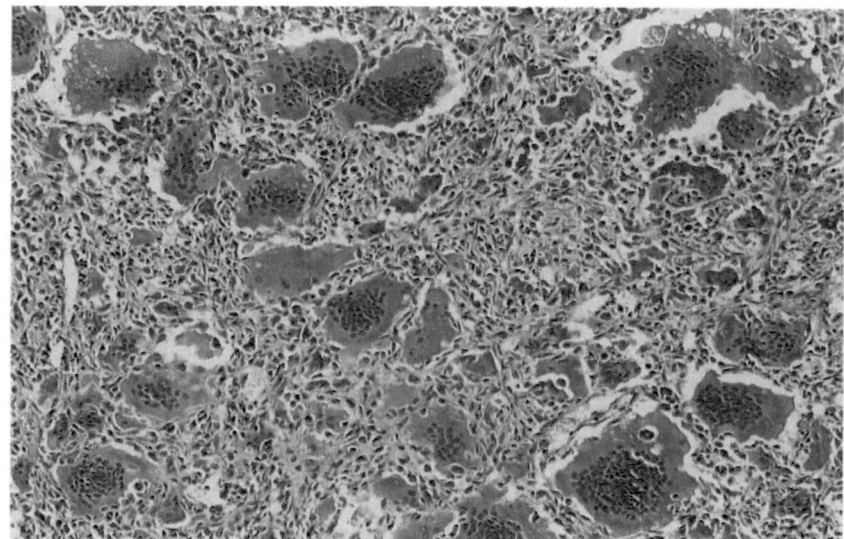

Fig. 89. *Giant-cell tumour.* Same case as Fig. 88

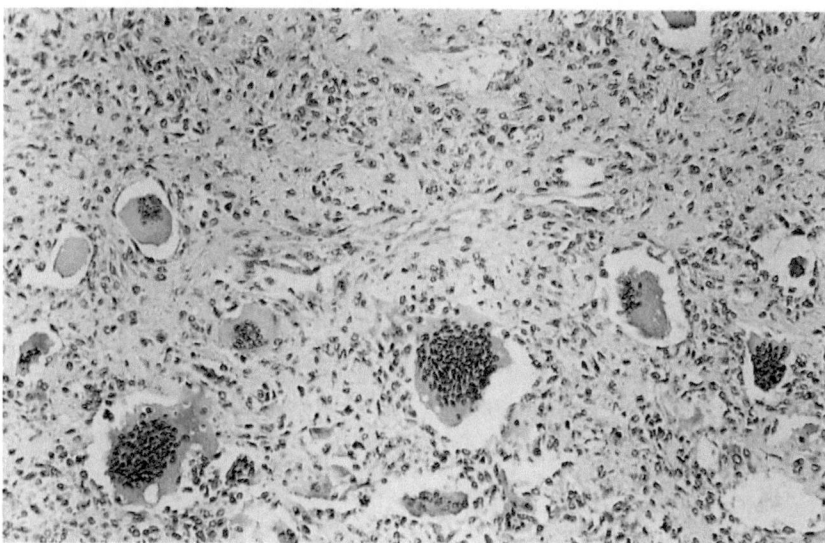

Fig. 90. *Giant-cell tumour.* Fibrous stroma

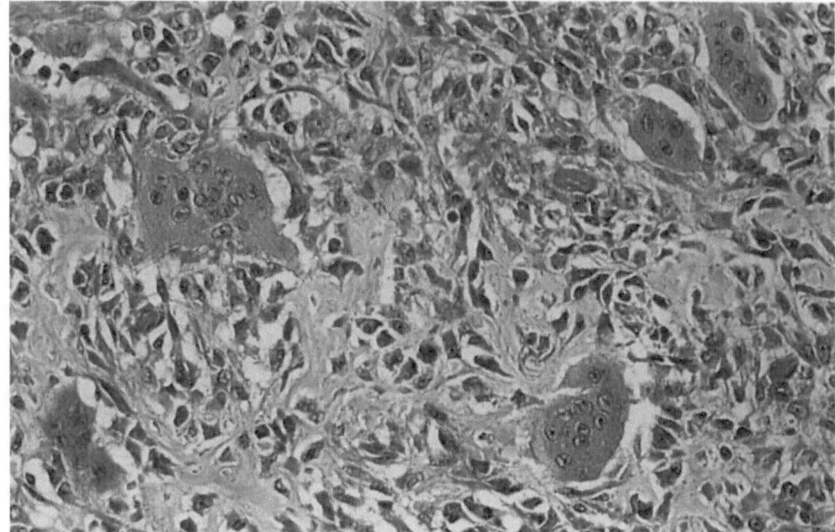

Fig. 91. *Giant-cell tumour.* Osteoid formation

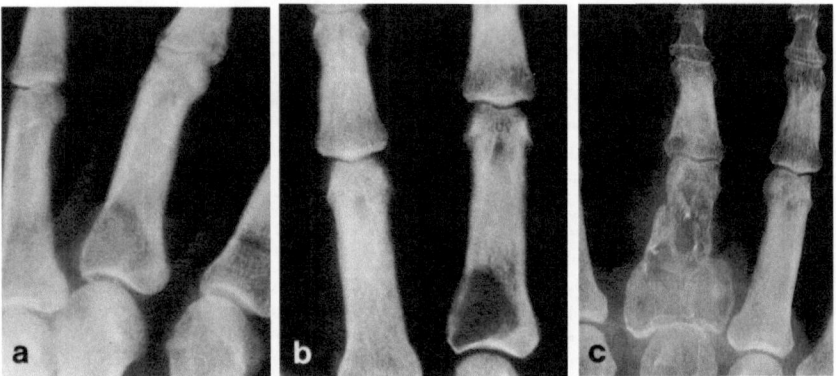

Fig. 92 a–c. *Giant-cell tumour.* Female, 46 years. Proximal phalanx of finger. **a, b** Radiographs (preoperative). **c** Radiograph (recurrence after curettage)

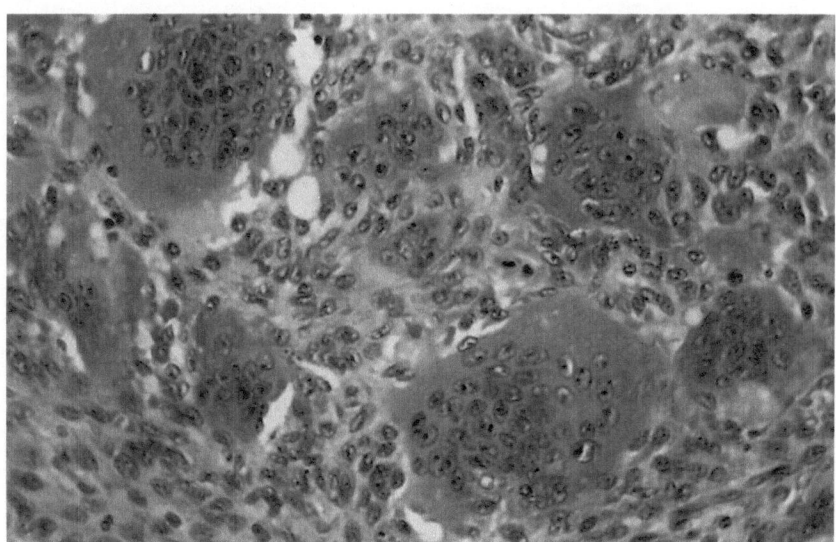

Fig. 93. *Giant-cell tumour.* Same case as Fig. 92. Original biopsy

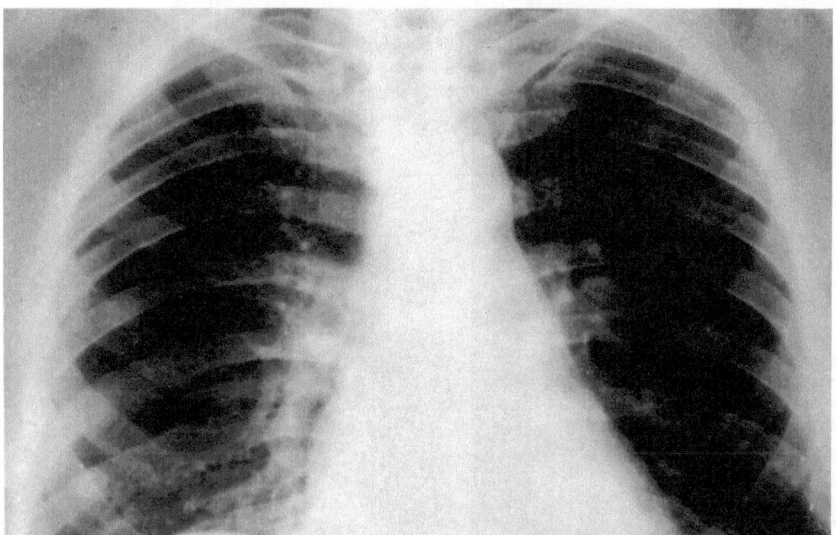

Fig. 94. *Giant-cell tumour.* Same case as Fig. 92. A metastasis is present in the lower lobe of the right lung. Radiograph

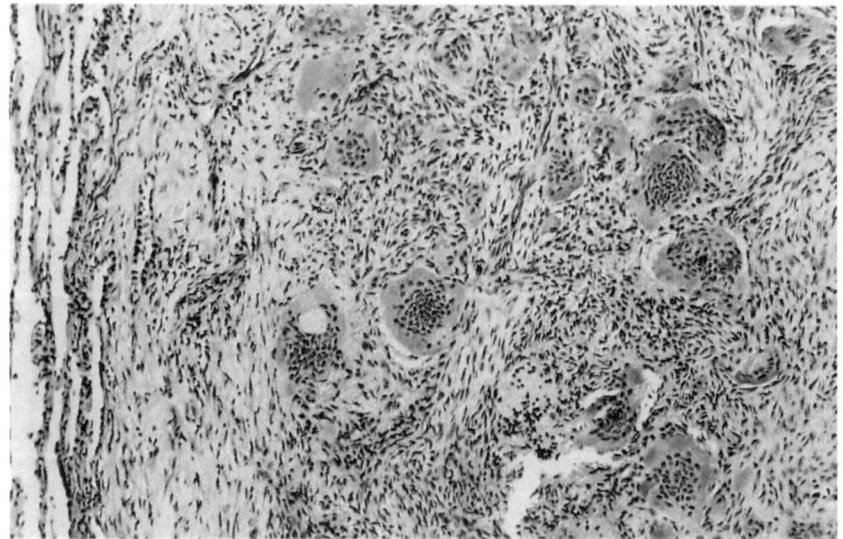

Fig. 95. *Giant-cell tumour.* Same case as Fig. 94. Histological appearance of excised pulmonary metastasis

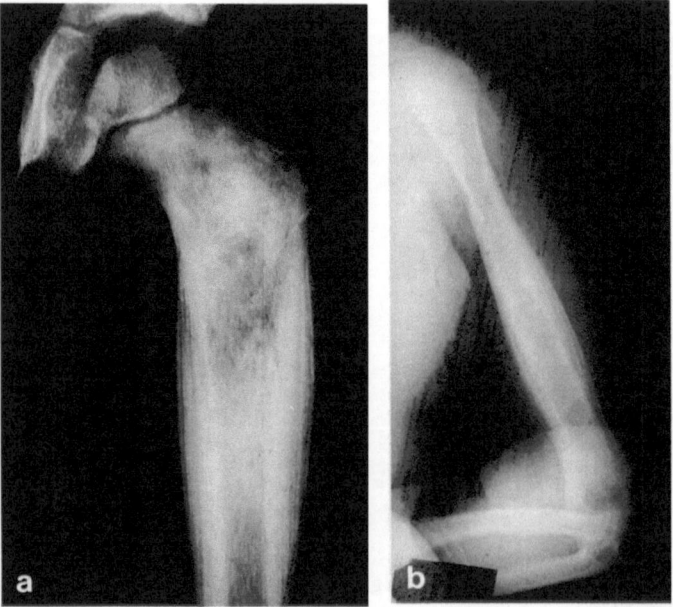

Fig. 96 a, b. *Ewing sarcoma.* Periosteal bone reactions. **a** Male, 5 years. Upper shaft of femur. Radiograph. **b** Male, 27 years. Shaft of humerus. Radiograph

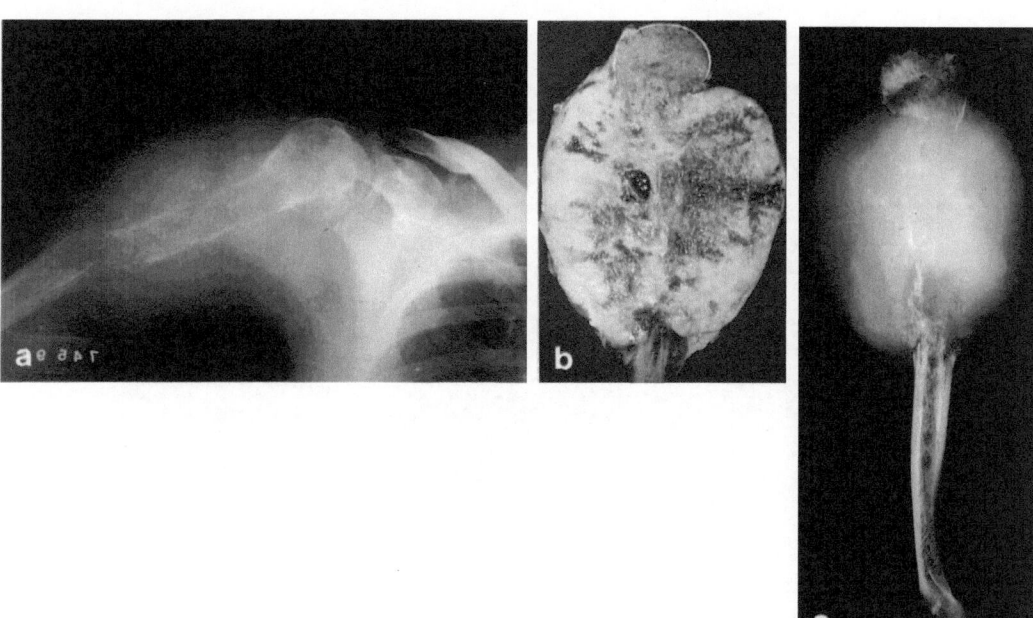

Fig. 97 a–c. *Ewing sarcoma.* Male, 25 years. Upper end of humerus. **a** Radiograph. **b** Photograph of specimen. **c** Radiograph of specimen

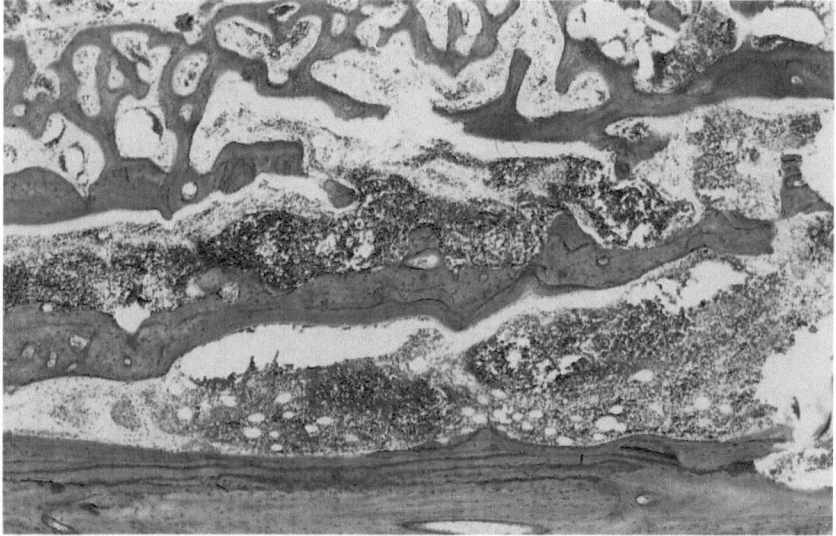

Fig. 98. *Ewing sarcoma.* Same case as Fig. 96 a. Periosteal reactive bone formation

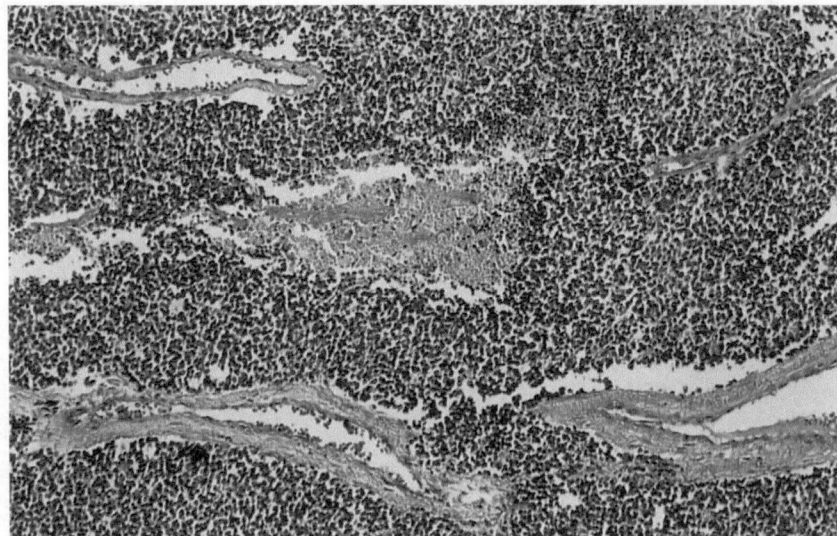

Fig. 99. *Ewing sarcoma.* Same case as Fig. 96 a

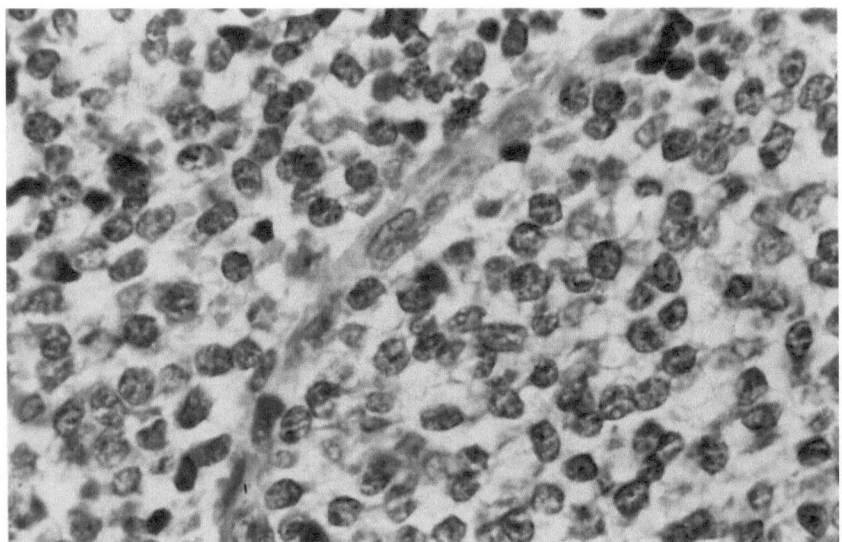

Fig. 100. *Ewing sarcoma.* Same case as Fig. 96 a

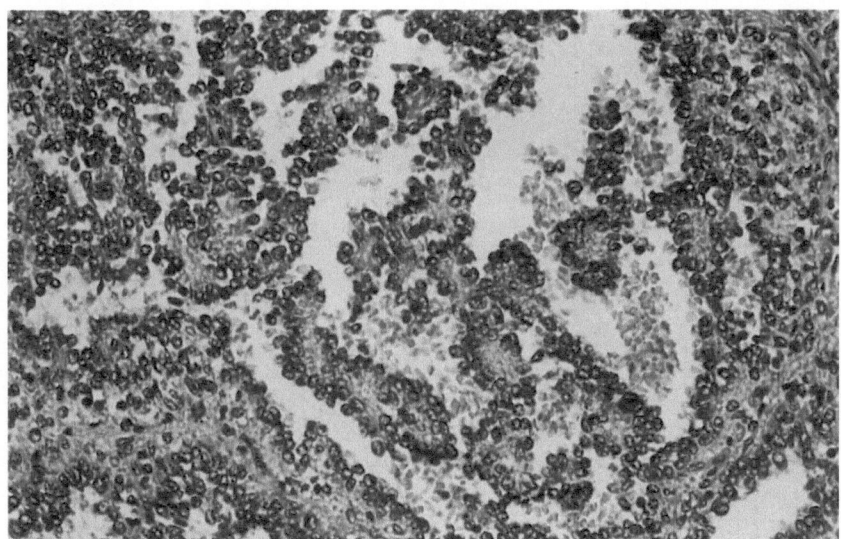

Fig. 101. *Ewing sarcoma*

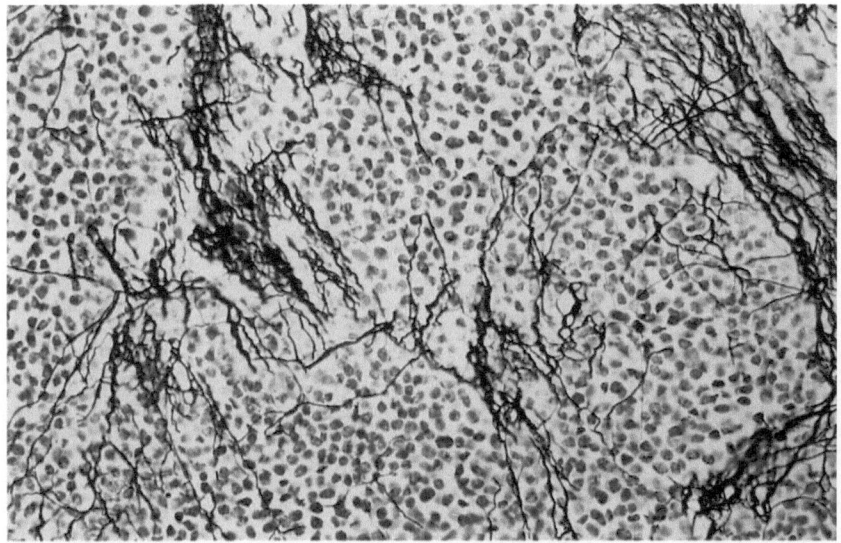

Fig. 102. *Ewing sarcoma.* Tumour divided into lobules by reticulin fibres

94

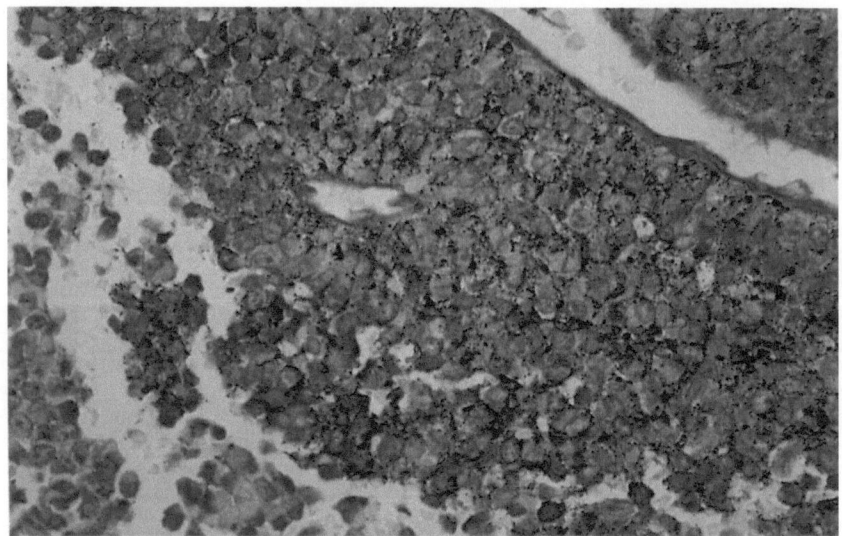

Fig. 103. *Ewing sarcoma.* Glycogen in cytoplasm of tumour cells. PAS

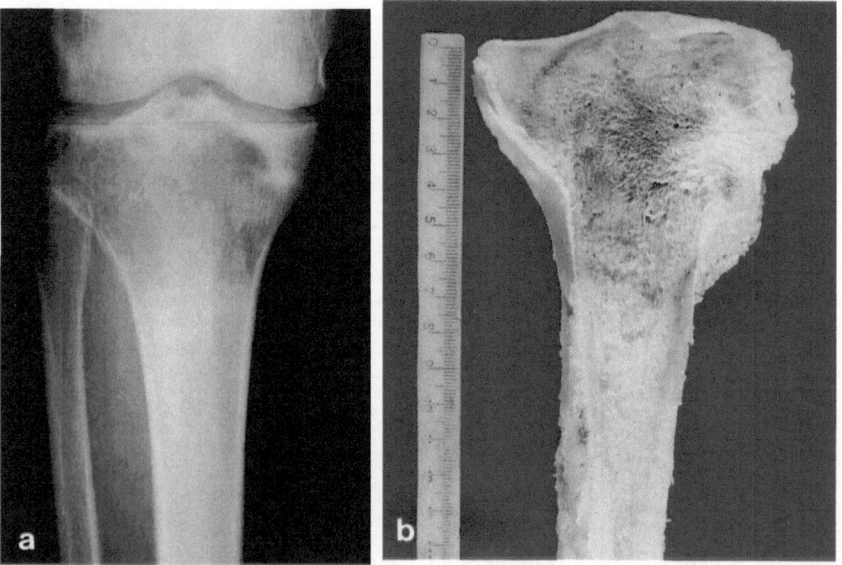

Fig. 104a, b. *Primitive neuroectodermal tumour of bone.* Male, 25 years. Upper end of tibia. **a** Radiograph. **b** Photograph of specimen

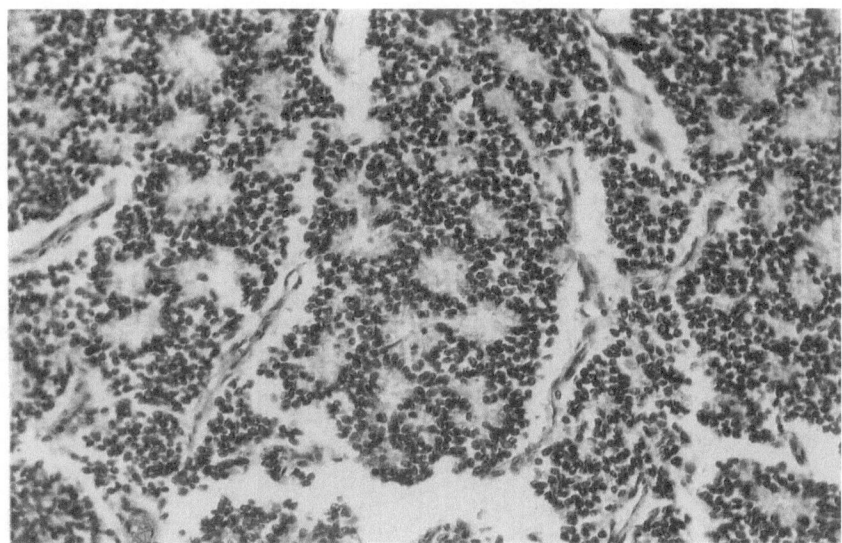

Fig. 105. *Primitive neuroectodermal tumour of bone.* Same case as Fig. 104. Prominent rosette formation

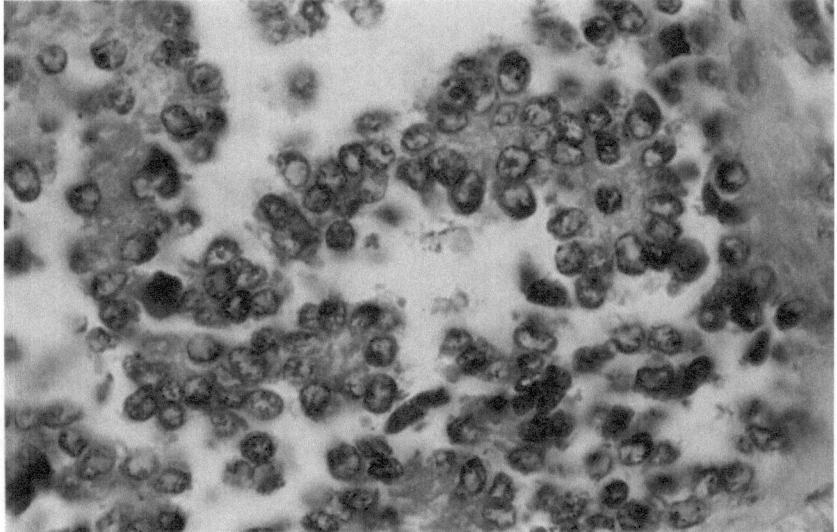

Fig. 106. *Primitive neuroectodermal tumour of bone.* Same case as Fig. 104

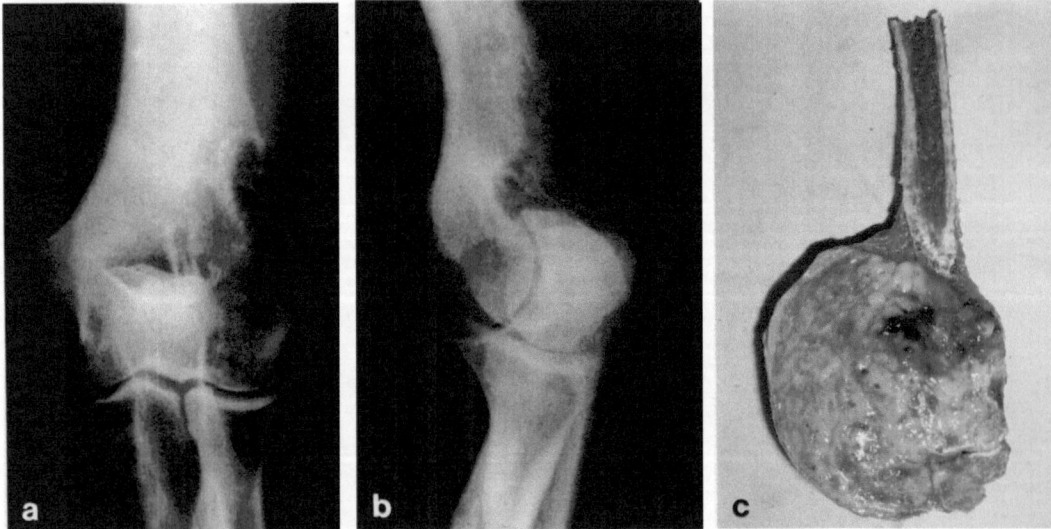

Fig. 107 a–c. *Malignant lymphoma of bone.* Male, 61 years. Lower end of humerus. **a, b** Radiographs. **c** Photograph of specimen

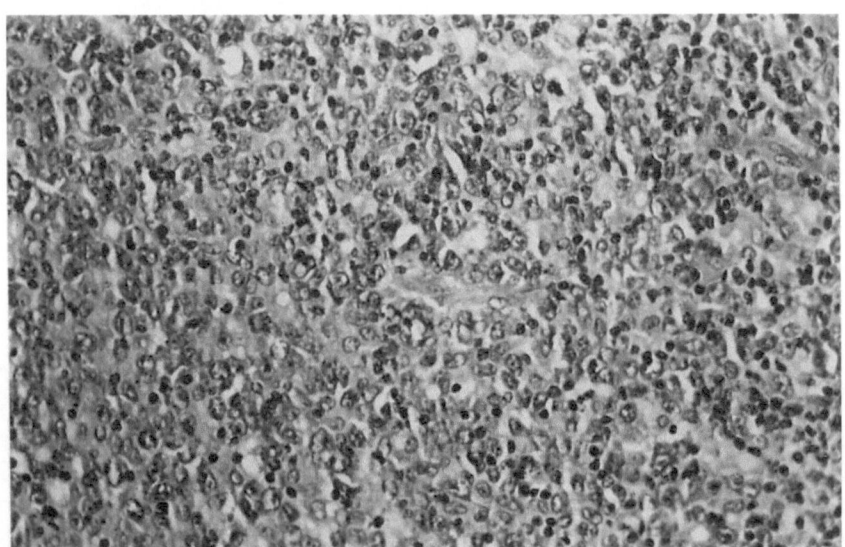

Fig. 108. *Malignant lymphoma of bone.* Same case as Fig. 107

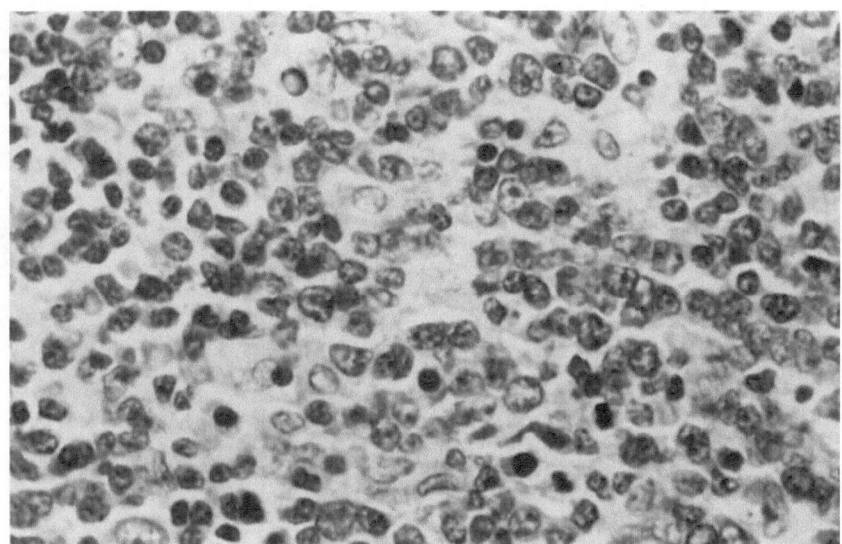

Fig. 109. *Malignant lymphoma of bone.* Large lymphoid cells

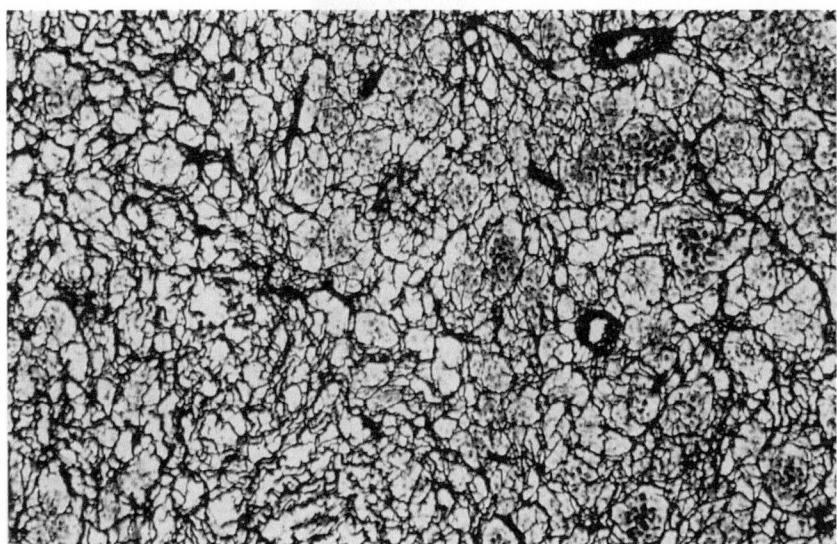

Fig. 110. *Malignant lymphoma of bone.* Same case as Fig. 107. Heavy reticulin fibre formation

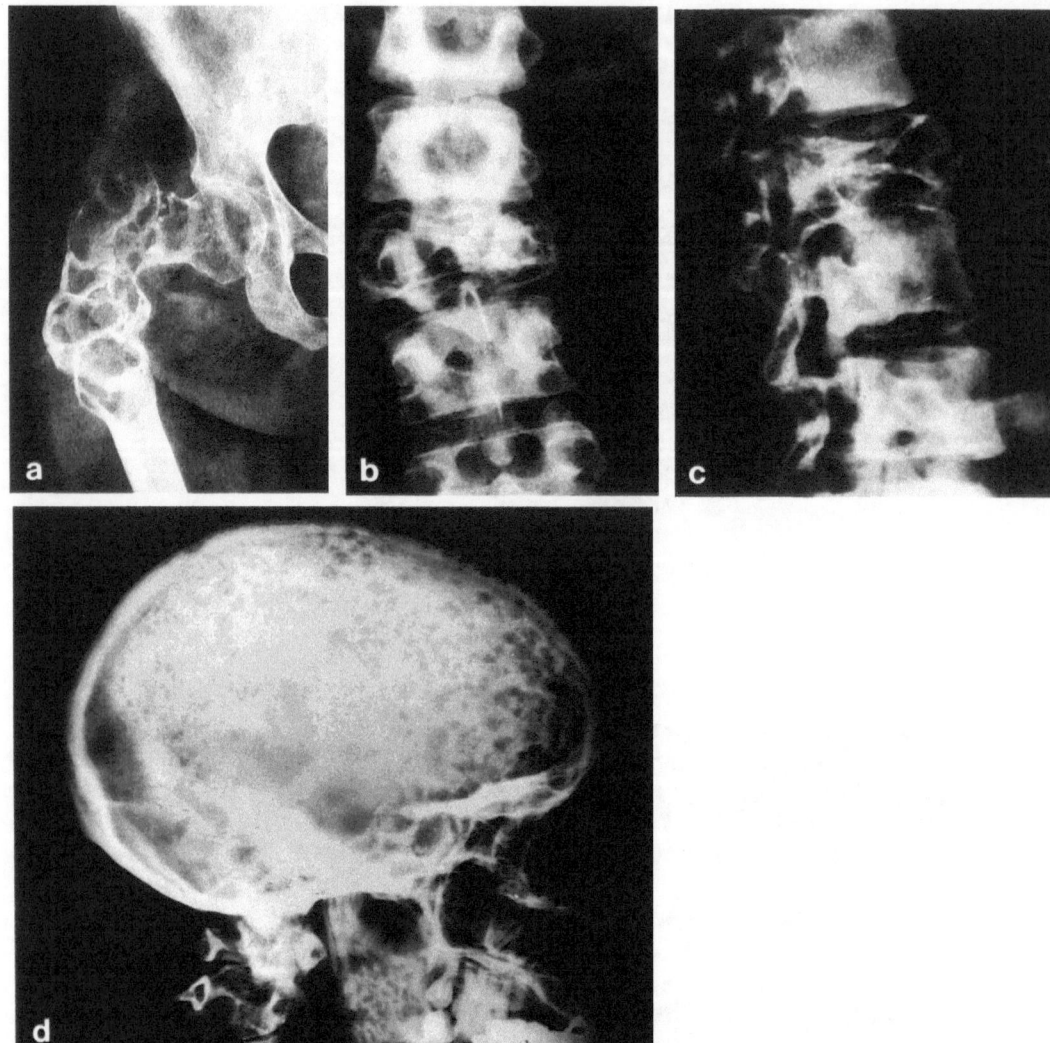

Fig. 111 a–d. *Myeloma.* Female, 42 years. Multiple lesions. Radiographs. **a** Upper femur, at time of presentation. **b, c** Lumbar spine, 2 years after presentation. **d** Skull, 3 years after presentation

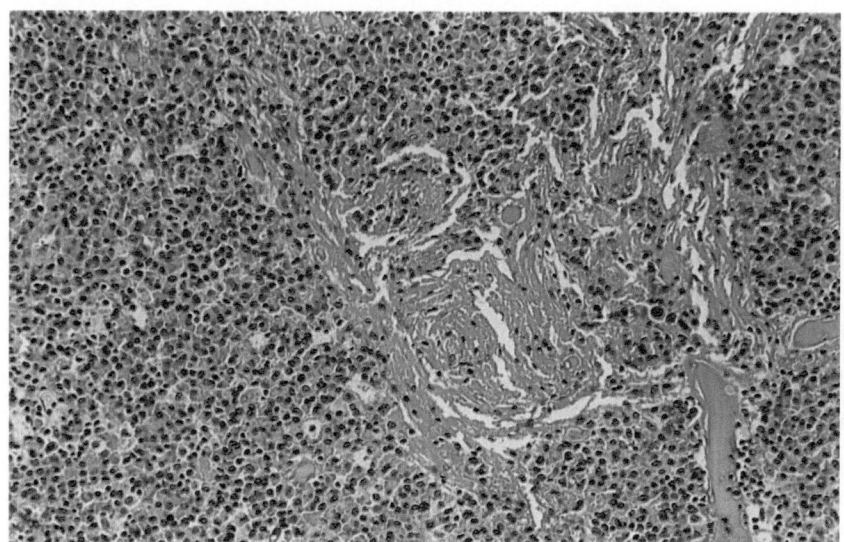

Fig. 112. *Myeloma.* Same case as Fig. 111

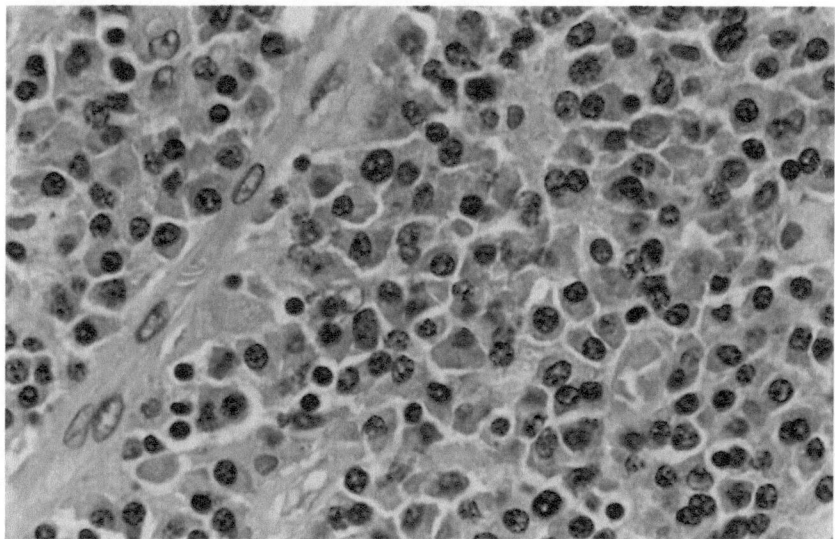

Fig. 113. *Myeloma.* Same case as Fig. 111

100

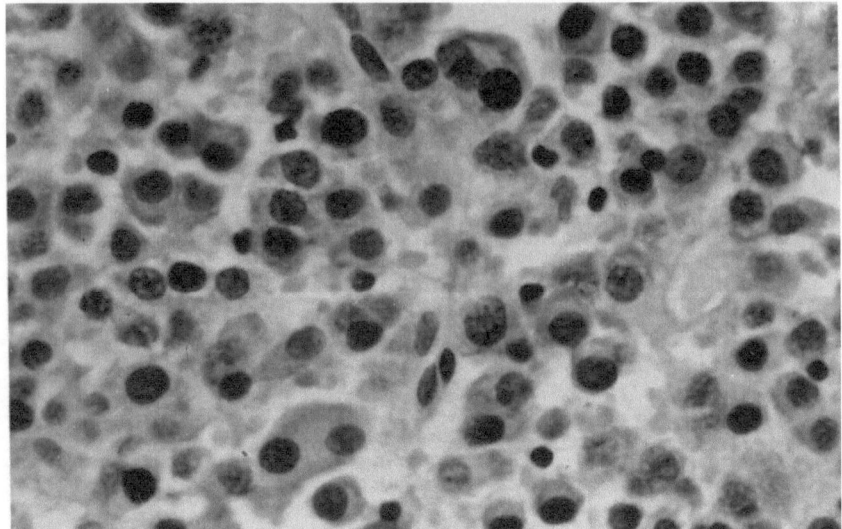

Fig. 114. *Myeloma.* Same case as Fig. 111

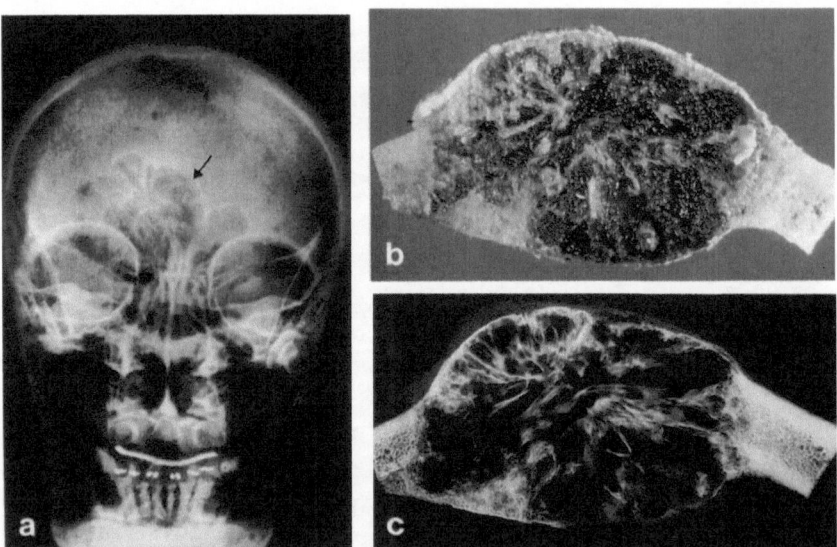

Fig. 115 a–c. *Haemangioma.* Female, 63 years. Frontal region of skull. **a** Radiograph. **b** Photograph of specimen. **c** Radiograph of specimen

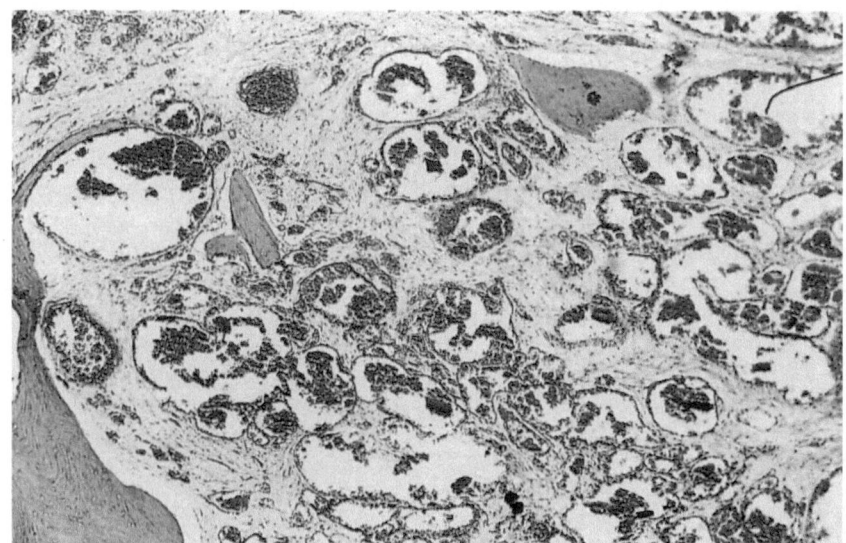

Fig. 116. *Haemangioma.* Same case as Fig. 115

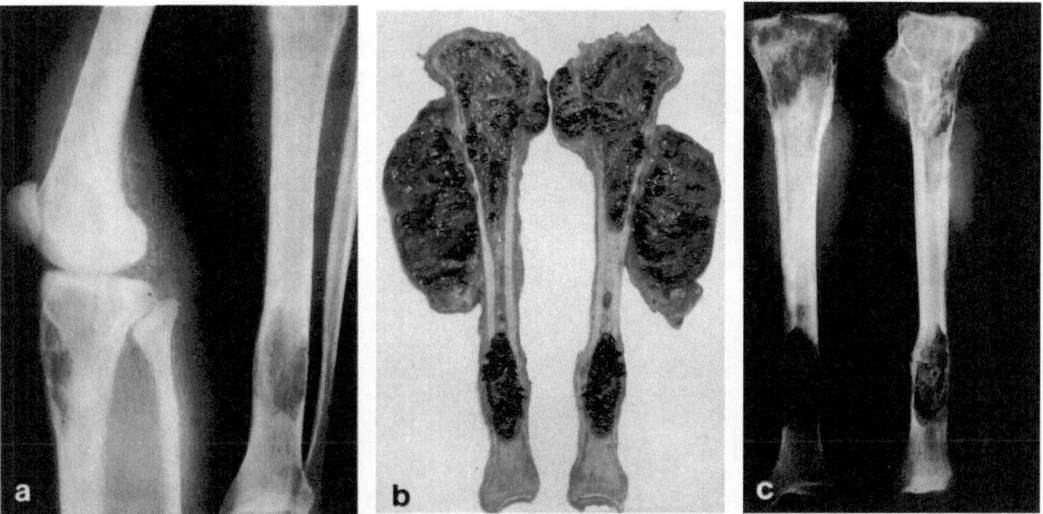

Fig. 117 a–c. *Haemangioendothelioma.* Male, 63 years. Multiple lesions of right tibia and femur. **a** Radiographs. **b** Photograph of specimen. **c** Radiograph of specimen

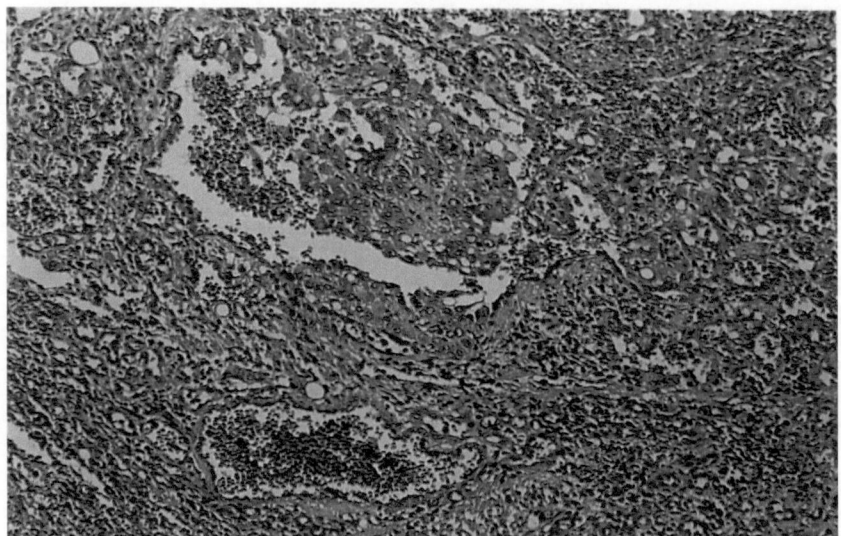

Fig. 118. *Haemangioendothelioma.* Same case as Fig. 117

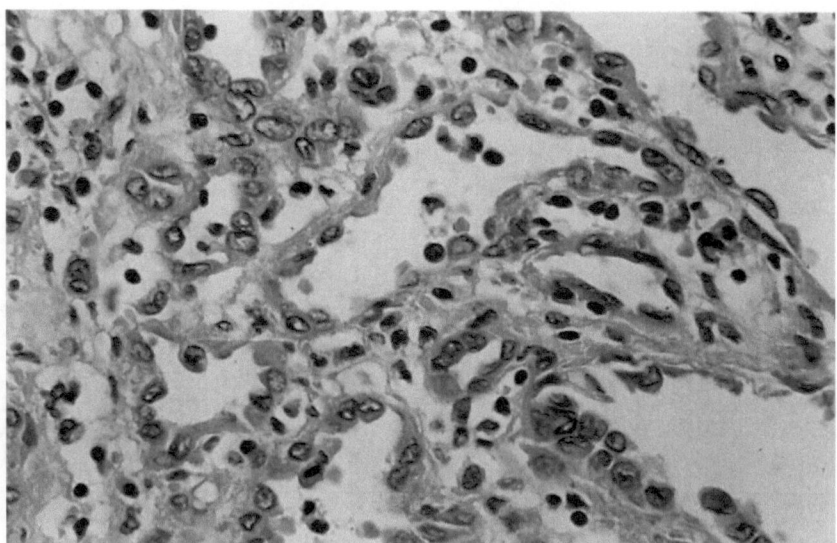

Fig. 119. *Haemangioendothelioma.* Same case as Fig. 117

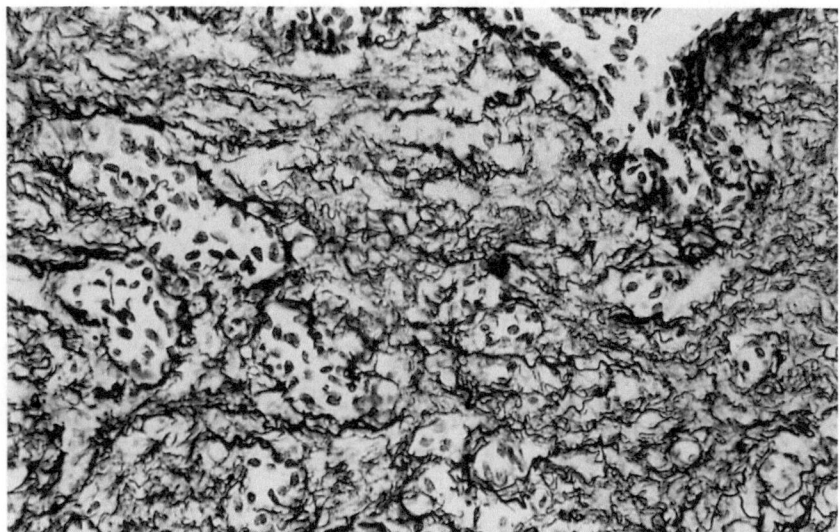

Fig. 120. *Haemangioendothelioma.* Same case as Fig. 117. Heavy reticulin fibre formation

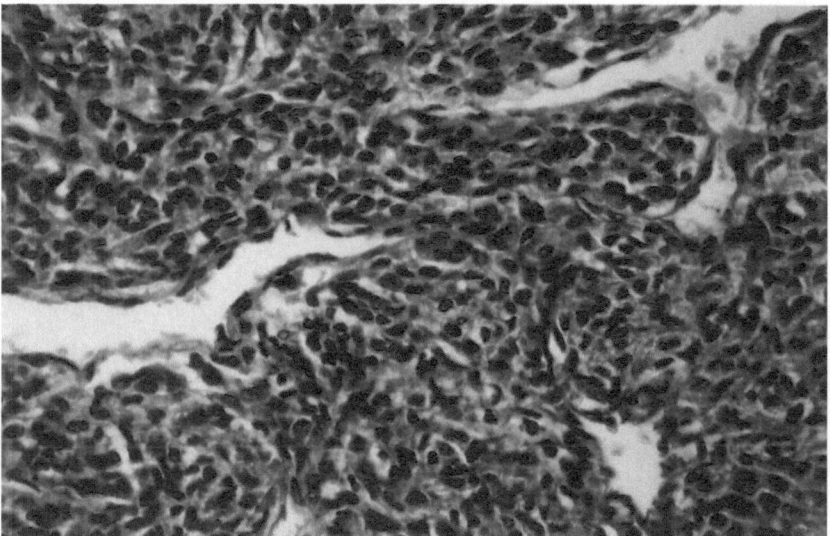

Fig. 121. *Haemangiopericytoma*

104

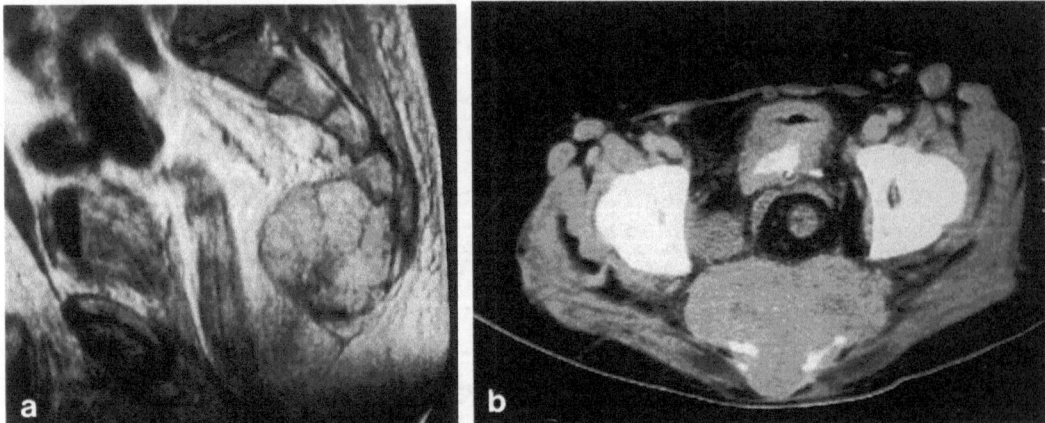

Fig. 122 a, b. *Angiosarcoma.* Male, 29 years. Sacrum. **a** Magnetic resonance image. **b** Tomogram

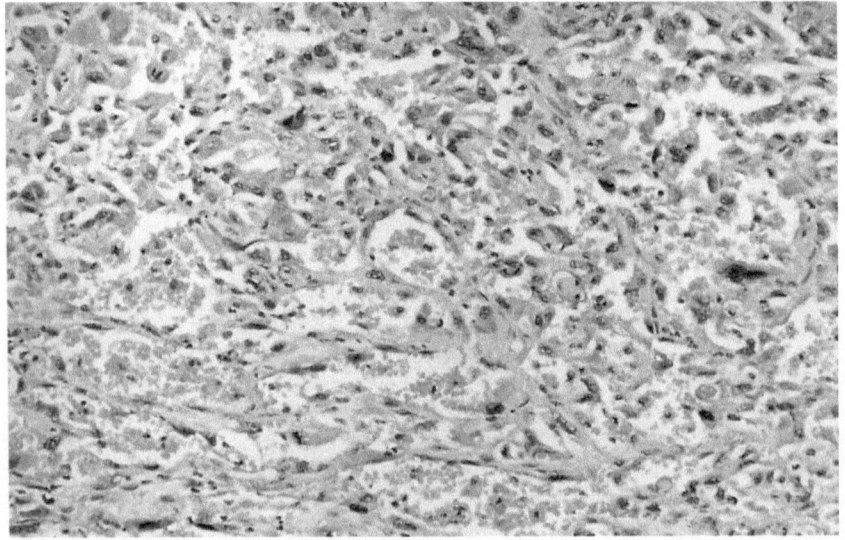

Fig. 123. *Angiosarcoma.* Same case as Fig. 122

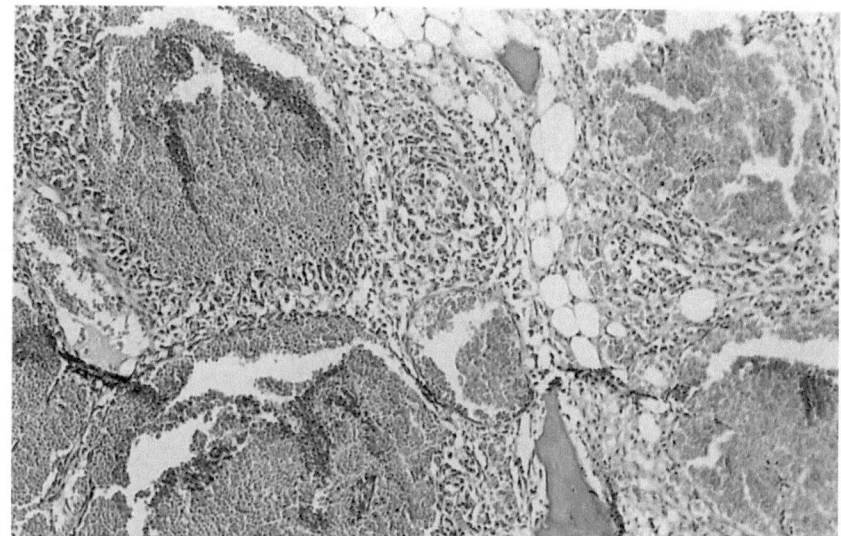

Fig. 124. *Angiosarcoma*

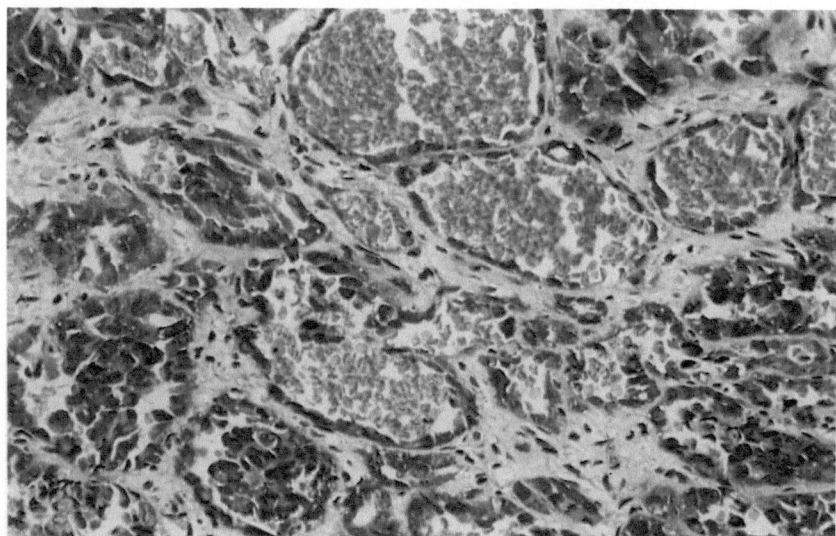

Fig. 125. *Angiosarcoma*

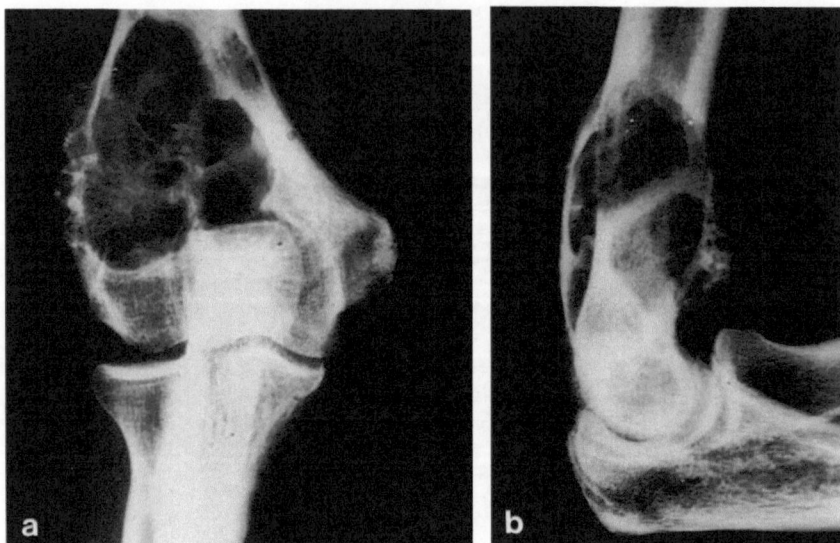

Fig. 126 a, b. *Desmoplastic fibroma.* Male, 56 years. Lower end of humerus. Radiographs

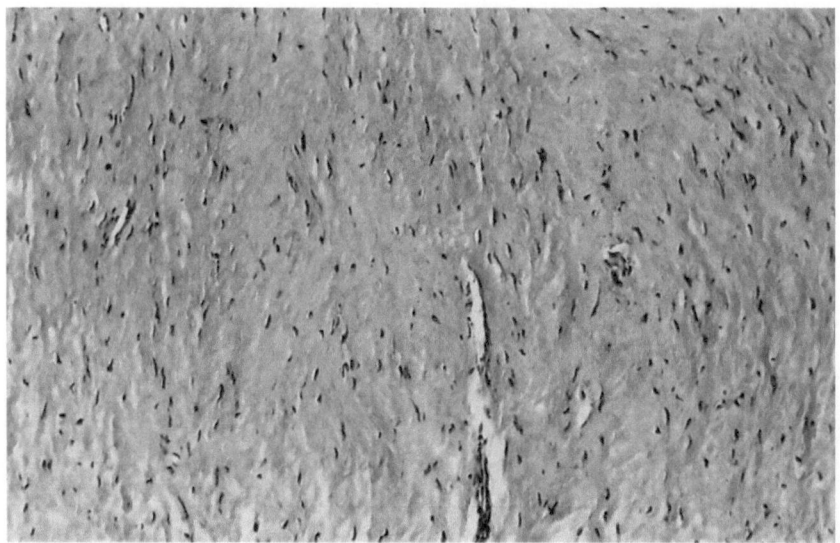

Fig. 127. *Desmoplastic fibroma.* Same case as Fig. 126

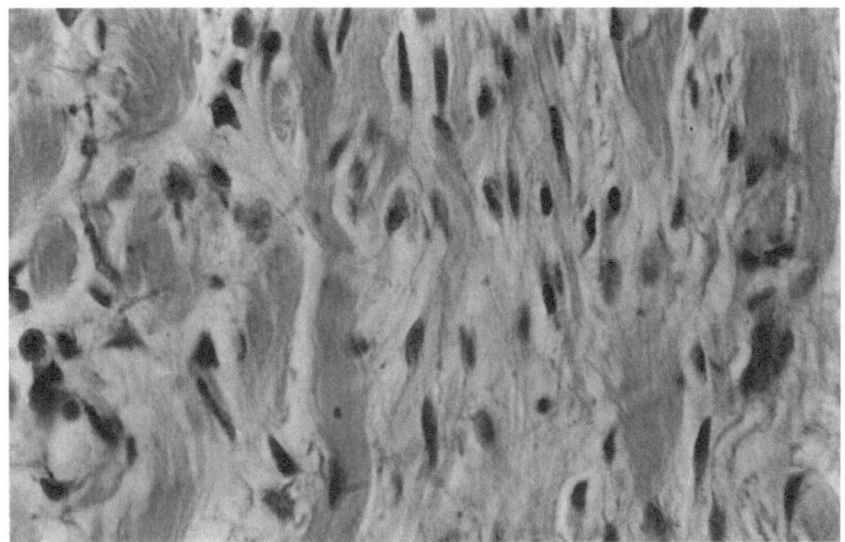

Fig. 128. *Desmoplastic fibroma.* Same case as Fig. 126

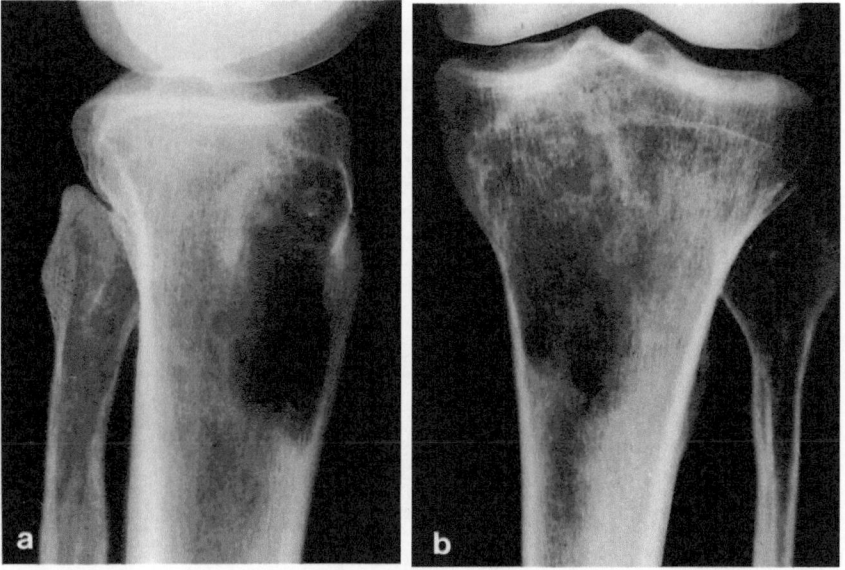

Fig. 129 a, b. *Fibrosarcoma.* Female, 67 years. Upper end of tibia. Radiographs

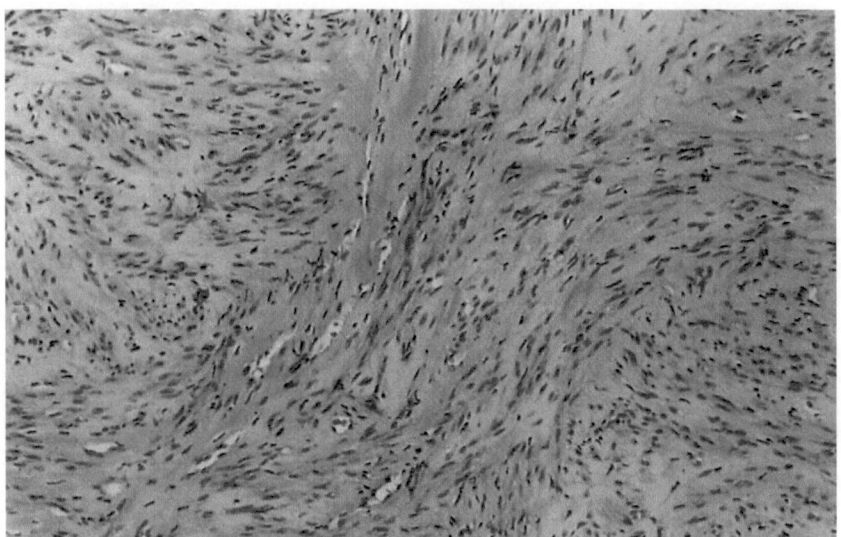

Fig. 130. *Fibrosarcoma.* Well-differentiated tumour

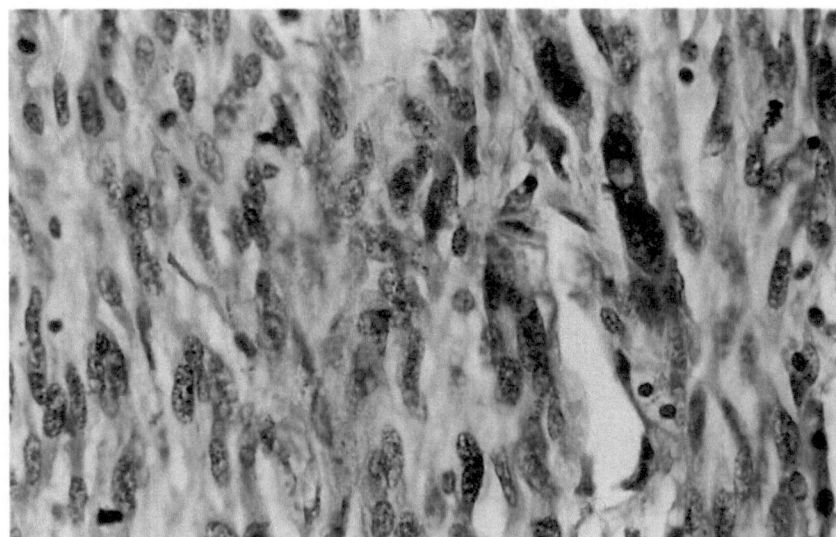

Fig. 131. *Fibrosarcoma.* Pleomorphic tumour

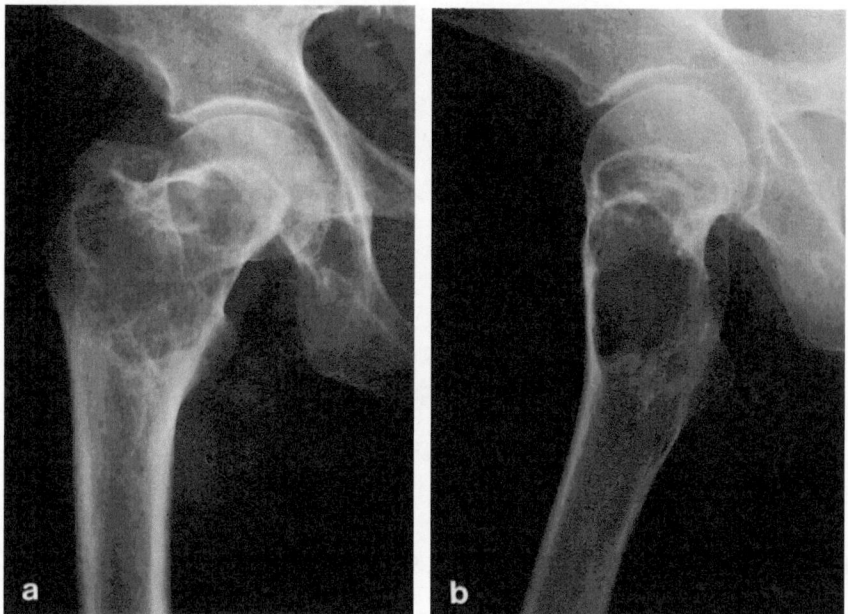

Fig. 132 a, b. *Malignant fibrous histiocytoma.* Female, 70 years. Upper end of femur. Radiographs

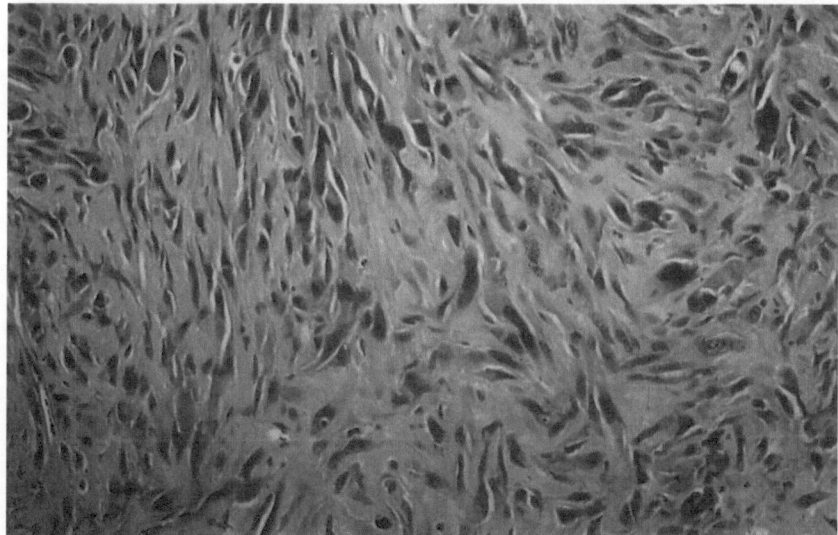

Fig. 133. *Malignant fibrous histiocytoma.* Same case as Fig. 132

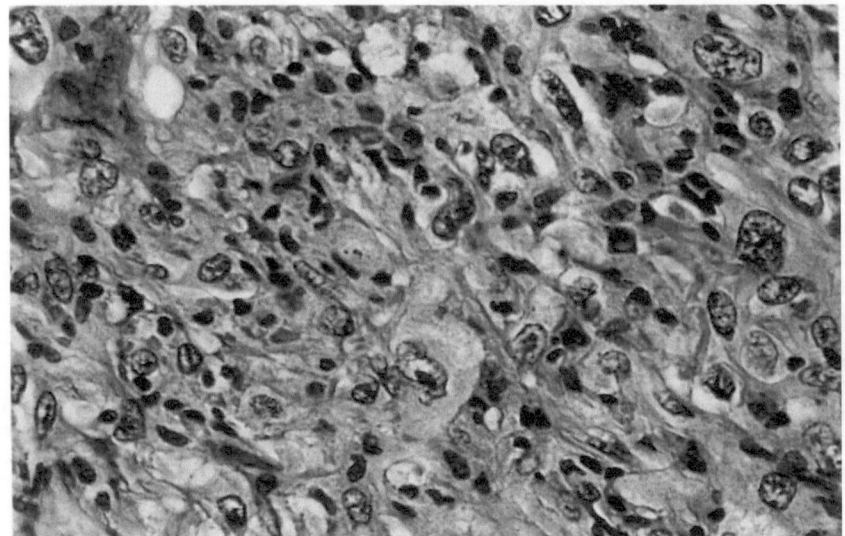

Fig. 134. *Malignant fibrous histiocytoma.* Same case as Fig. 132

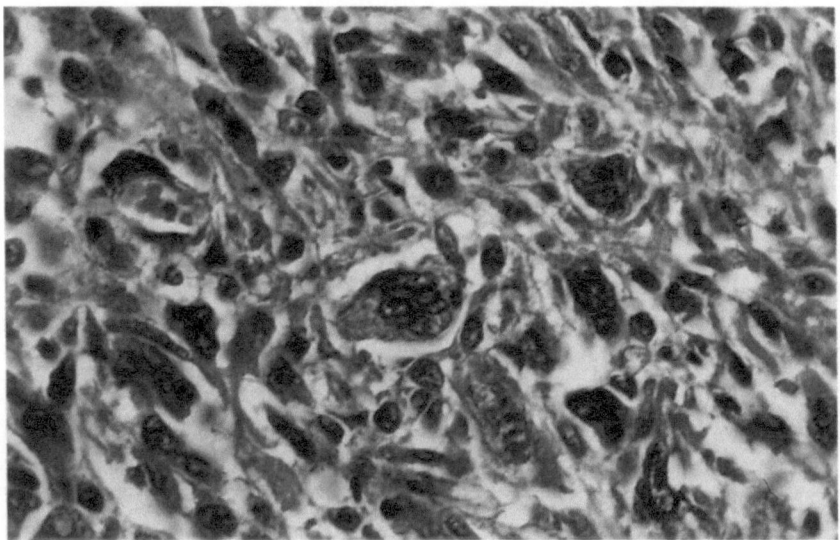

Fig. 135. *Malignant fibrous histiocytoma.* Same case as Fig. 132

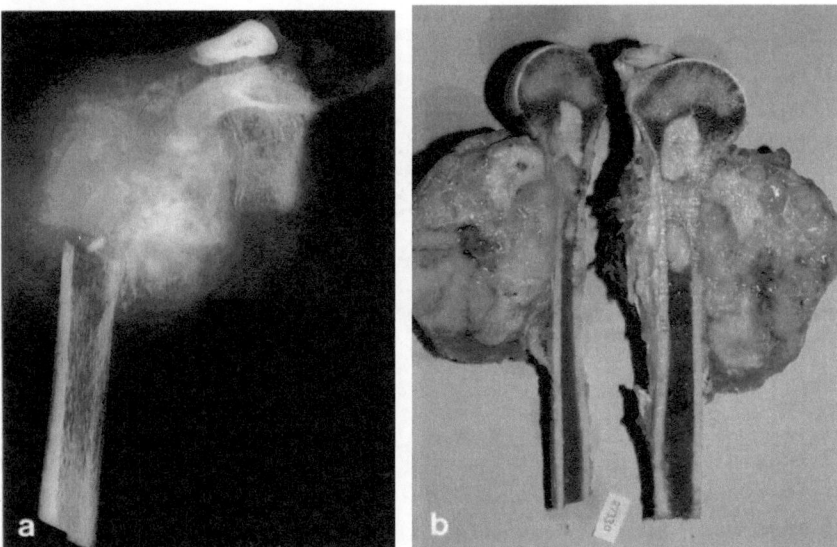

Fig. 136 a, b. *Malignant mesenchymoma.* Female, 32 years. Upper end of humerus. **a** Radiograph. **b** Photograph of specimen

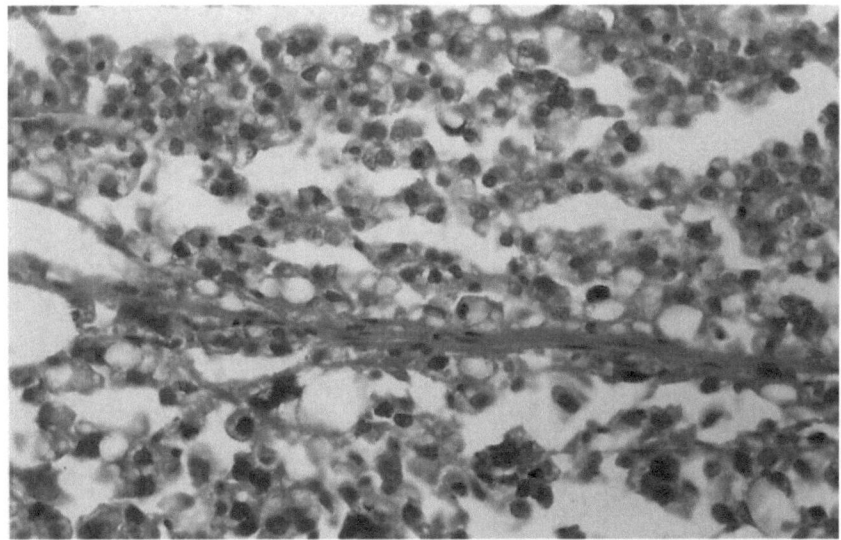

Fig. 137. *Malignant mesenchymoma.* Liposarcomatous pattern. Same case as Fig. 136

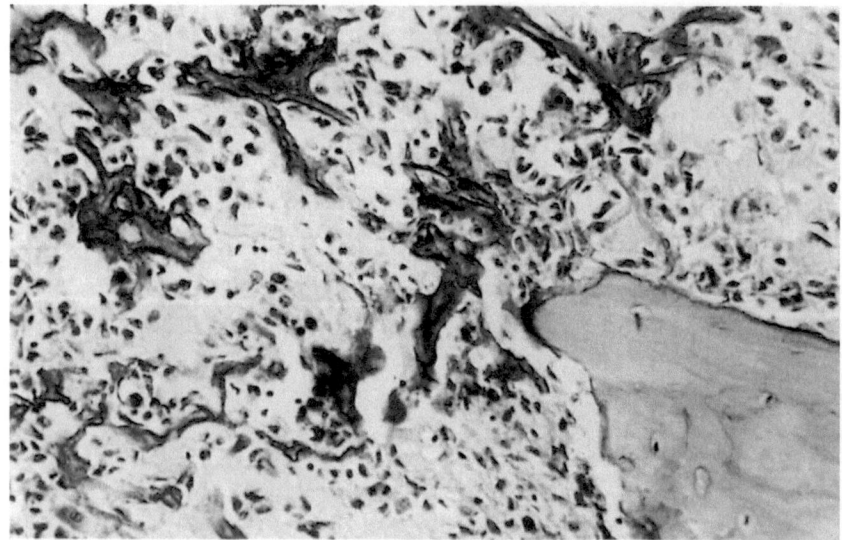

Fig. 138. *Malignant mesenchymoma.* Osteosarcomatous pattern. Same case as Fig. 136

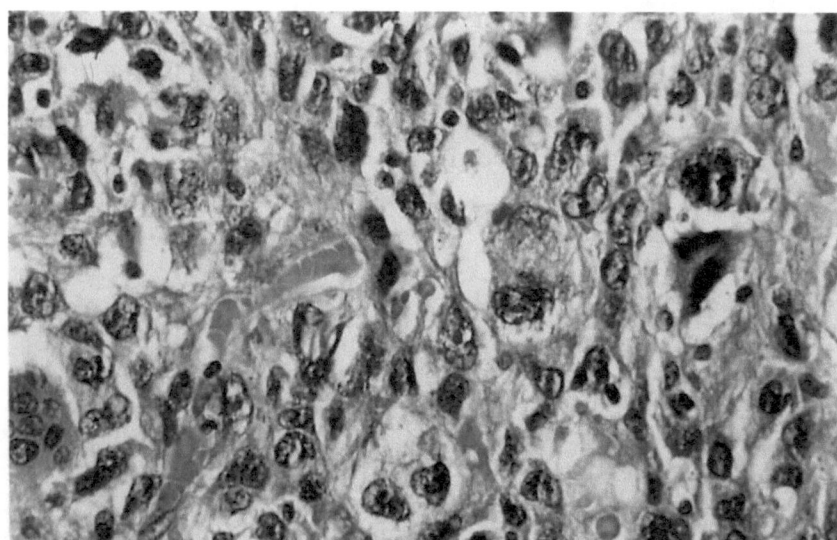

Fig. 139. *Undifferentiated sarcoma*

113

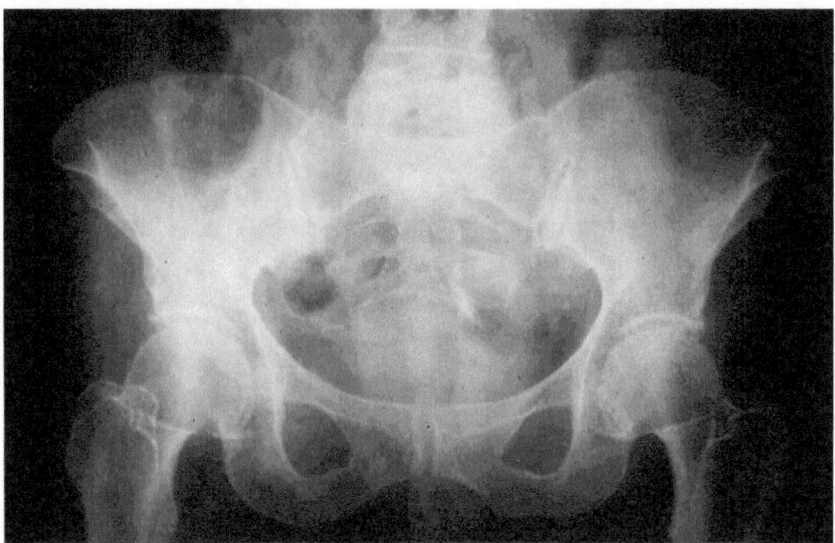

Fig. 140. *Chordoma.* Female, 62 years. Sacrum. Radiograph

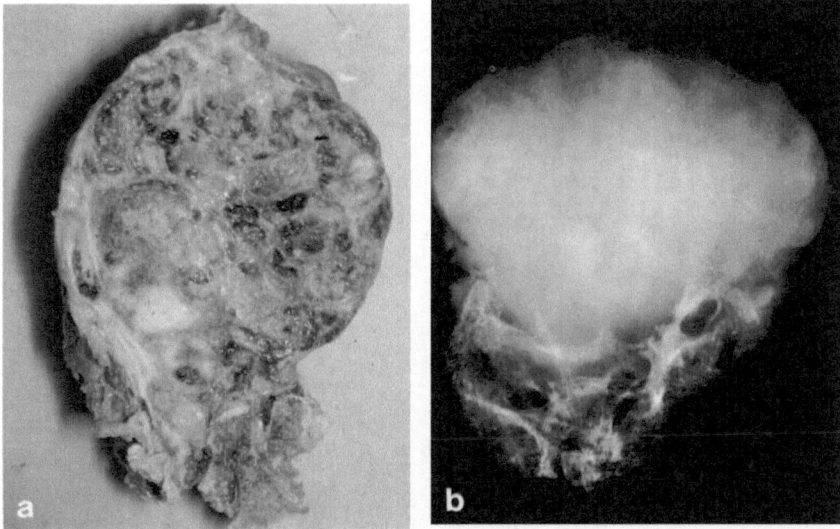

Fig. 141 a, b. *Chordoma.* Same case as Fig. 140. **a** Photograph of specimen.
b Radiograph of specimen

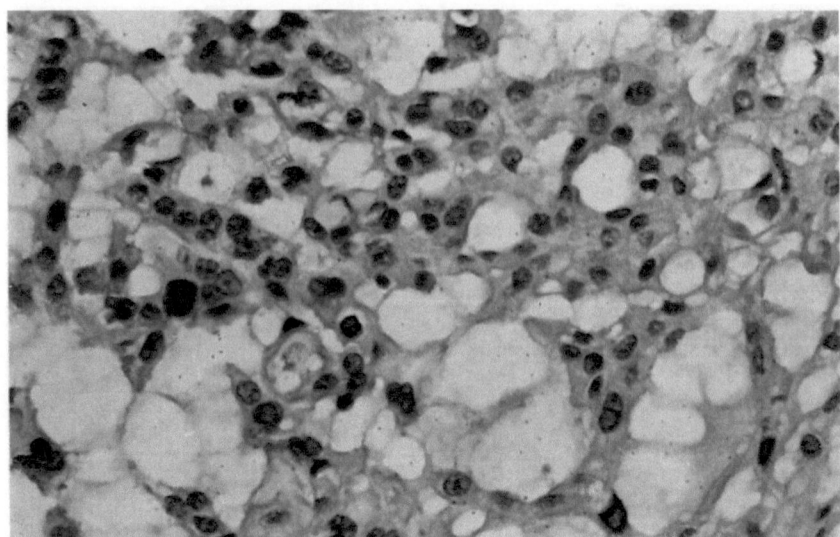

Fig. 142. *Chordoma.* Same case as Fig. 140

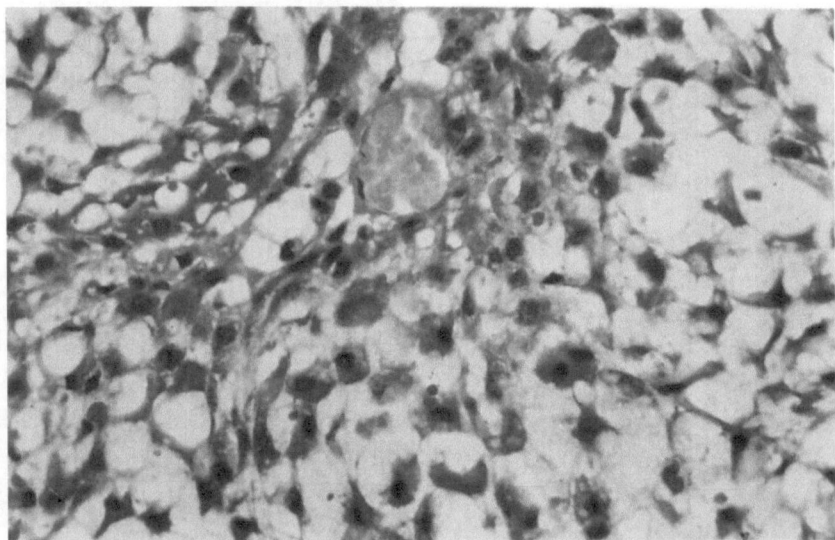

Fig. 143. *Chordoma.* Same case as Fig. 140. Glycogen in cytoplasm of tumour cells. PAS

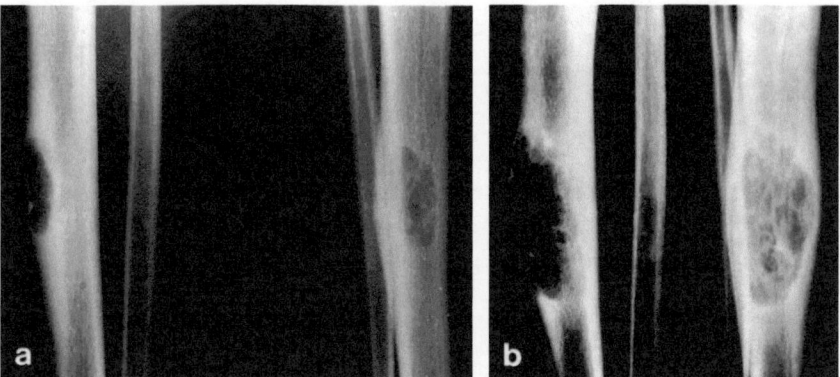

Fig. 144a, b. *Adamantinoma of long bones.* Male, 12 years. Shaft of tibia. **a** Radiographs (initial presentation). **b** Radiographs (1 year after curettage)

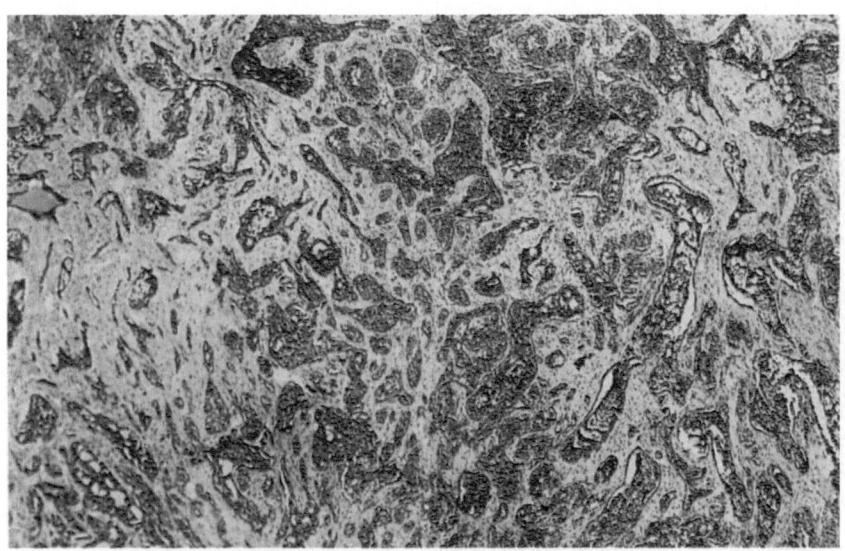

Fig. 145 *Adamantinoma of long bones.* Same case as Fig. 144

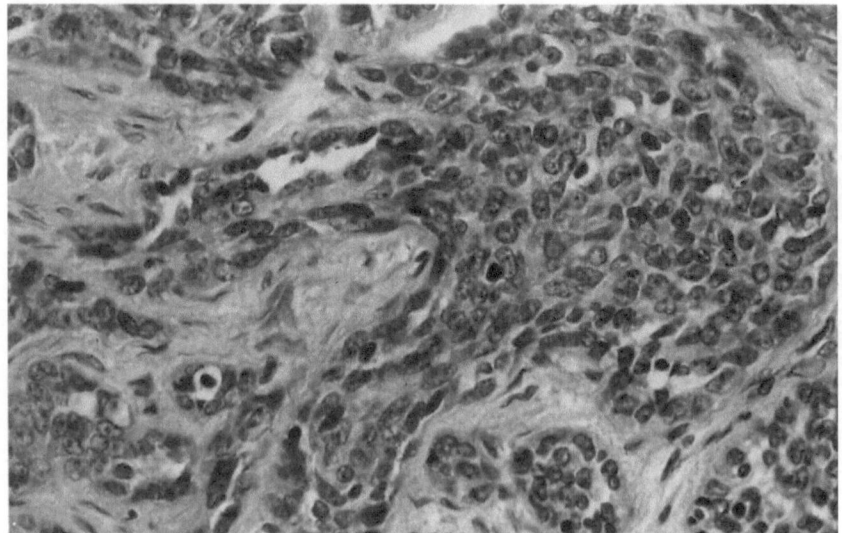

Fig. 146. *Adamantinoma of long bones*

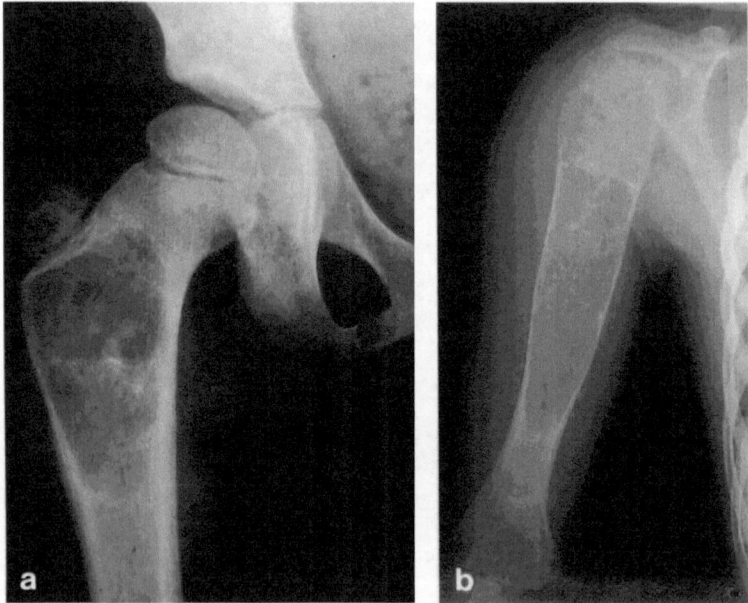

Fig. 147 a, b. *Solitary bone cyst.* **a** Female, 8 years. Upper shaft of femur. Radiograph. **b** Female, 6 years. Upper shaft of humerus. Radiograph

117

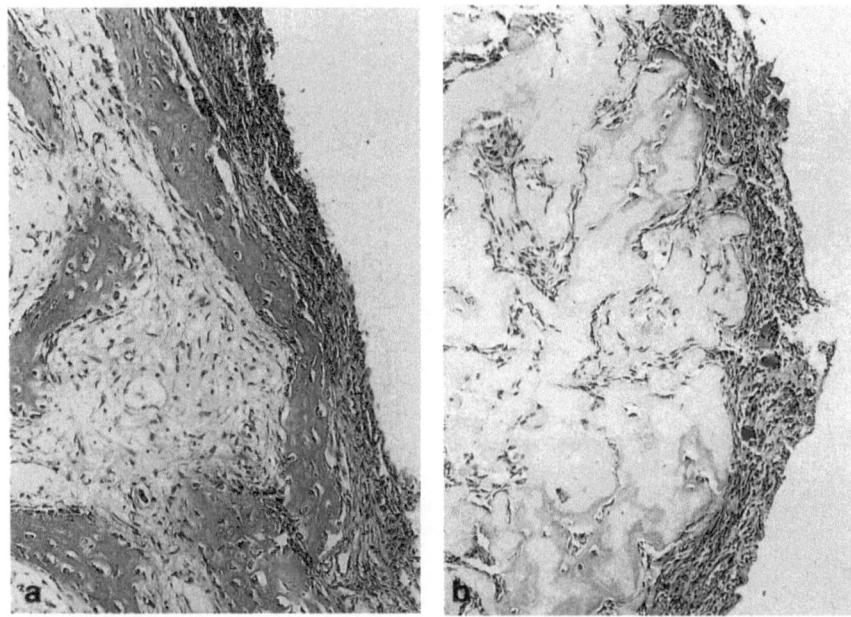

Fig. 148 a,b. *Solitary bone cyst*

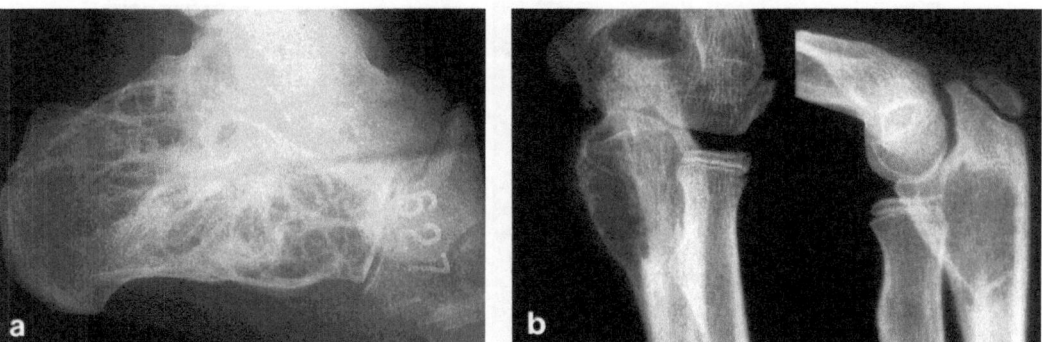

Fig. 149 a,b. *Aneurysmal bone cyst.* **a** Male, 35 years. Calcaneus. Radiograph. **b** Female, 10 years. Metaphysis of ulna. Radiograph

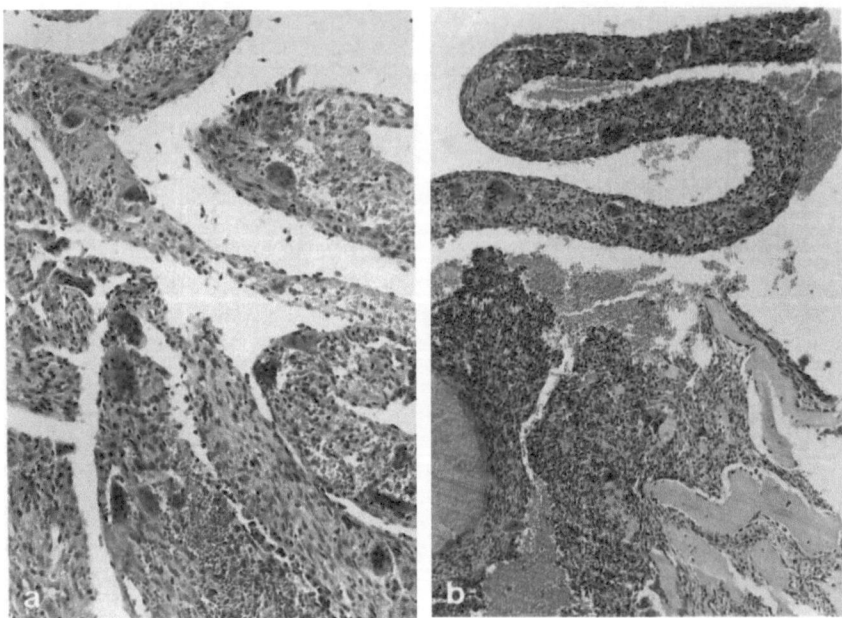

Fig. 150. *Aneurysmal bone cyst*

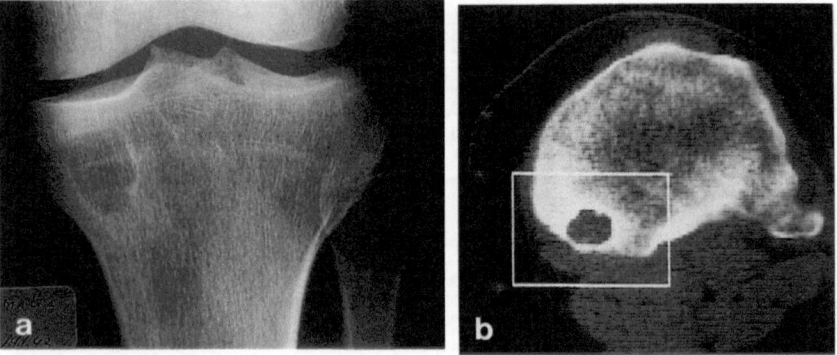

Fig. 151 a, b. *Juxta-articular bone cyst.* Female, 48 years. Upper end of tibia.
a Radiograph. **b** Tomogram

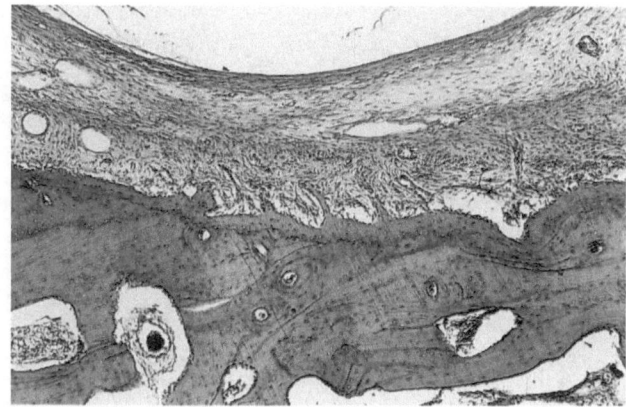

Fig. 152. *Juxta-articular bone cyst*

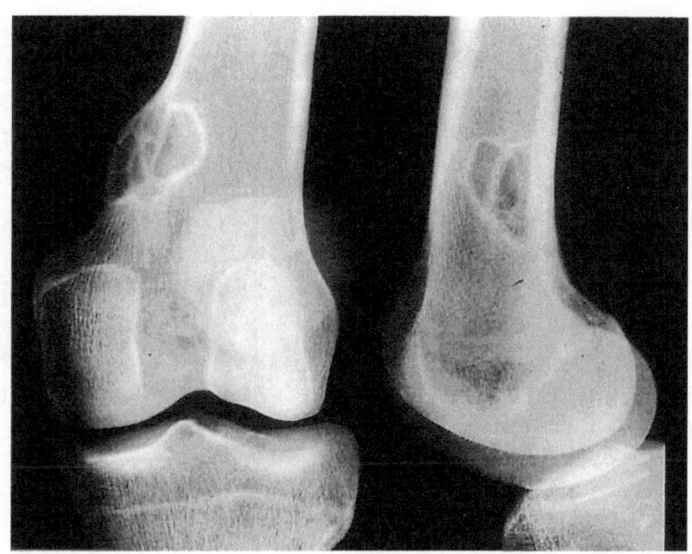

Fig. 153. *Metaphyseal fibrous defect.* Female, 15 years. Lower metaphysis of femur. Radiograph

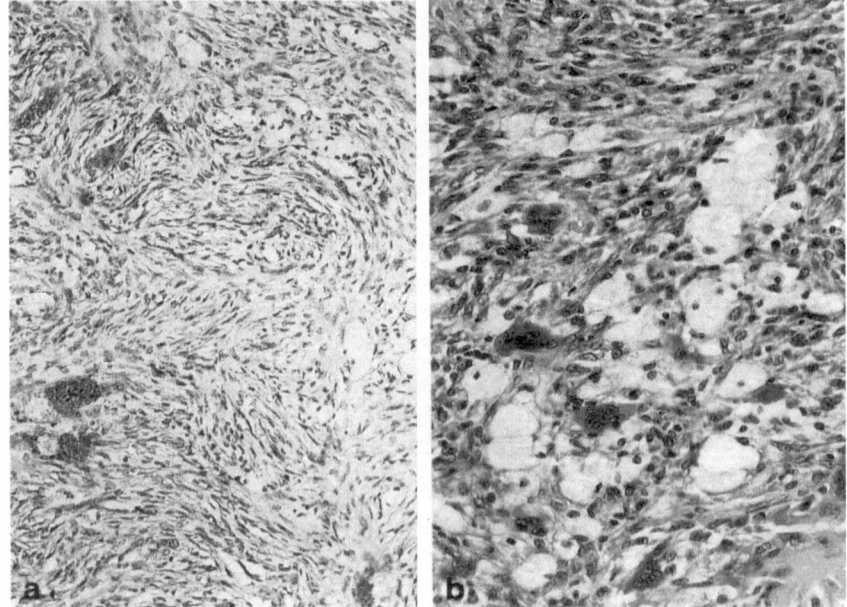

Fig. 154 a, b. *Metaphyseal fibrous defect*

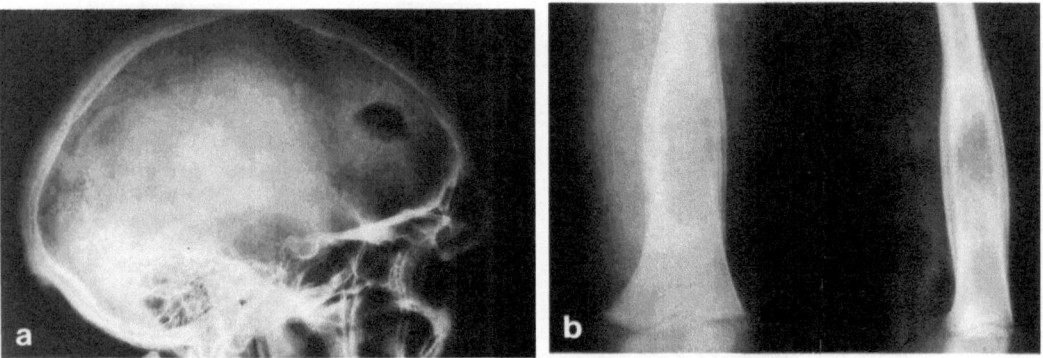

Fig. 155 a, b. *Eosinophilic granuloma.* **a** Male, 20 years. Frontal bone. Radiograph. **b** Male, 6 years. Shaft of femur. Radiograph

121

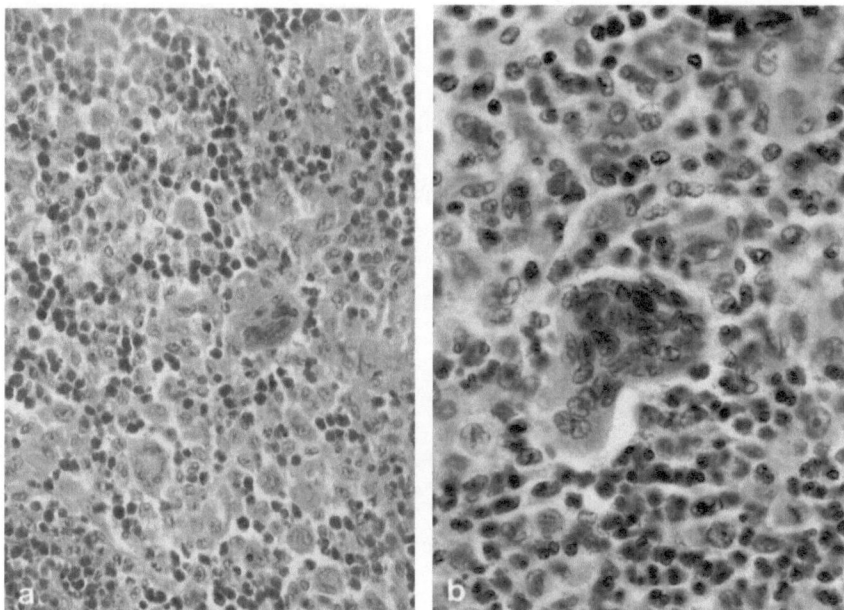

Fig. 156 a, b. *Eosinophilic granuloma*

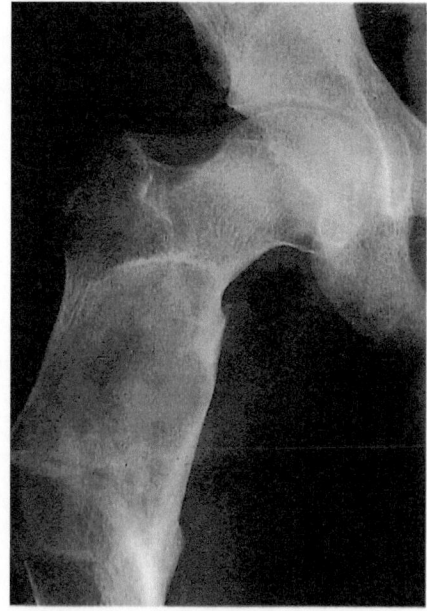

Fig. 157. *Fibrous dysplasia.* Female, 14 years. Upper shaft of femur. Radiograph

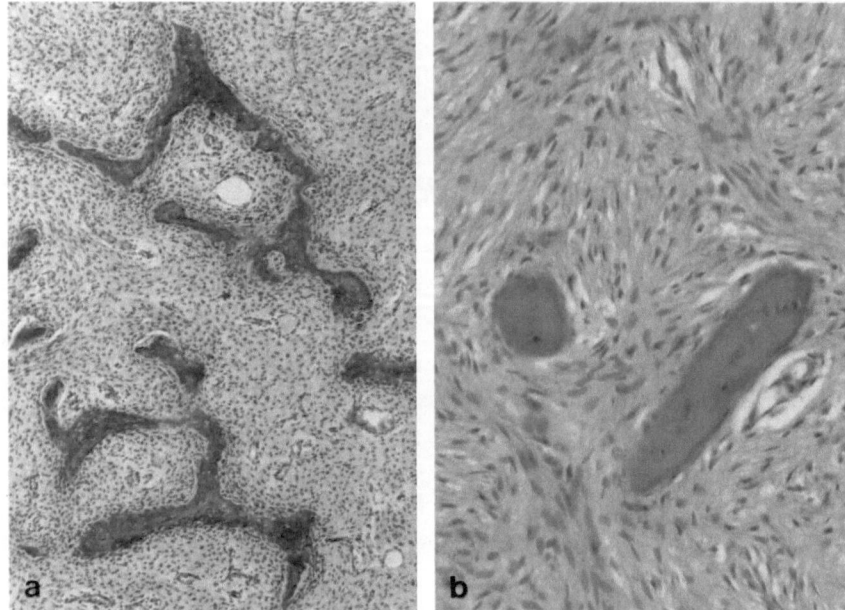

Fig. 158 a, b. *Fibrous dysplasia*

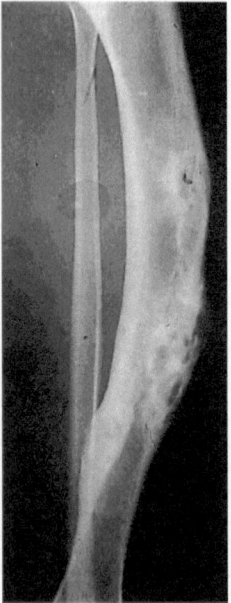

Fig. 159. *Osteofibrous dysplasia.* Male, 6 years. Shaft of tibia. Radiograph

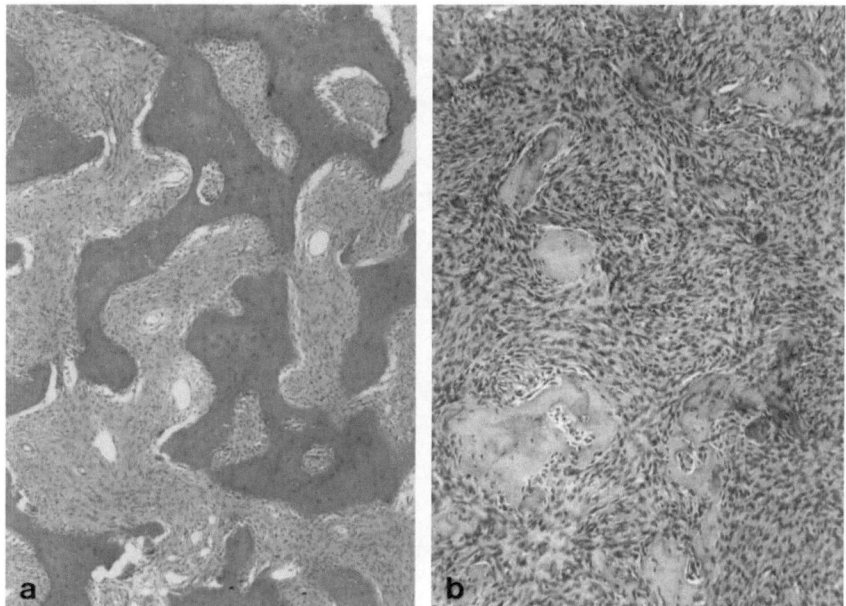

Fig. 160 a, b. *Osteofibrous dysplasia*

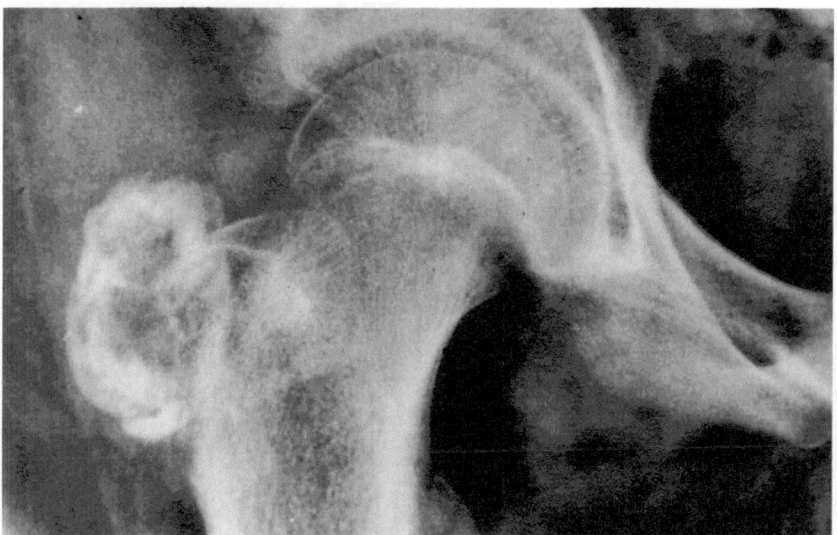

Fig. 161. *Myositis ossificans*. Male, 13 years. Soft tissues of trochanteric region. Radiograph

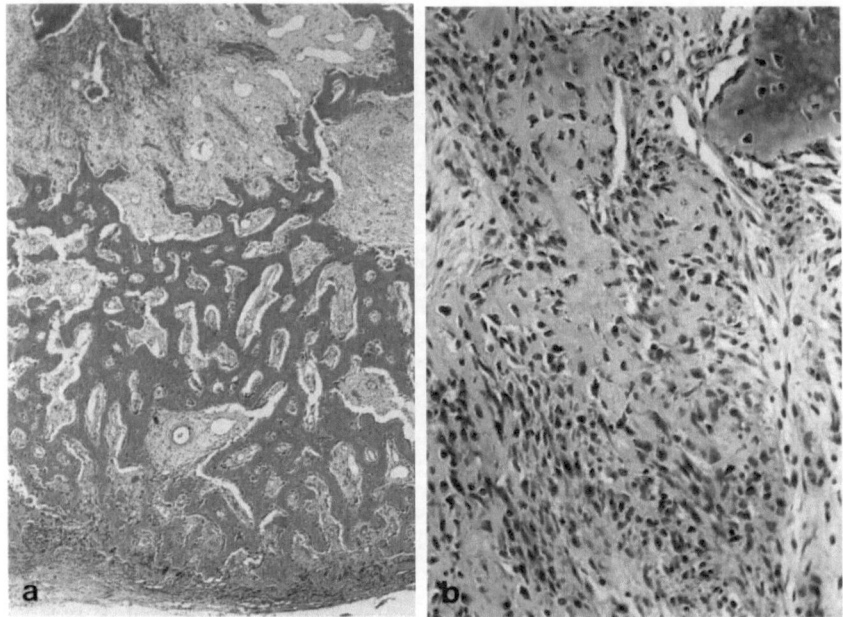

Fig. 162 a, b. *Myositis ossificans.* Same case as Fig. 161

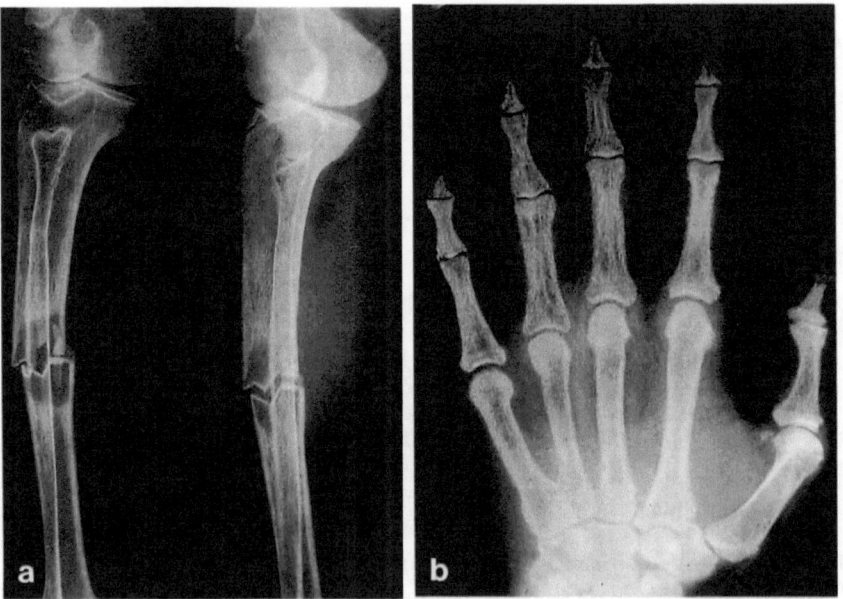

Fig. 163 a, b. *Brown tumour of hyperparathyroidism.* Female, 60 years. Multiple bone lesions, parathyroid adenoma removed. **a** Tibia and fibula. Radiograph. **b** Hand. Radiograph

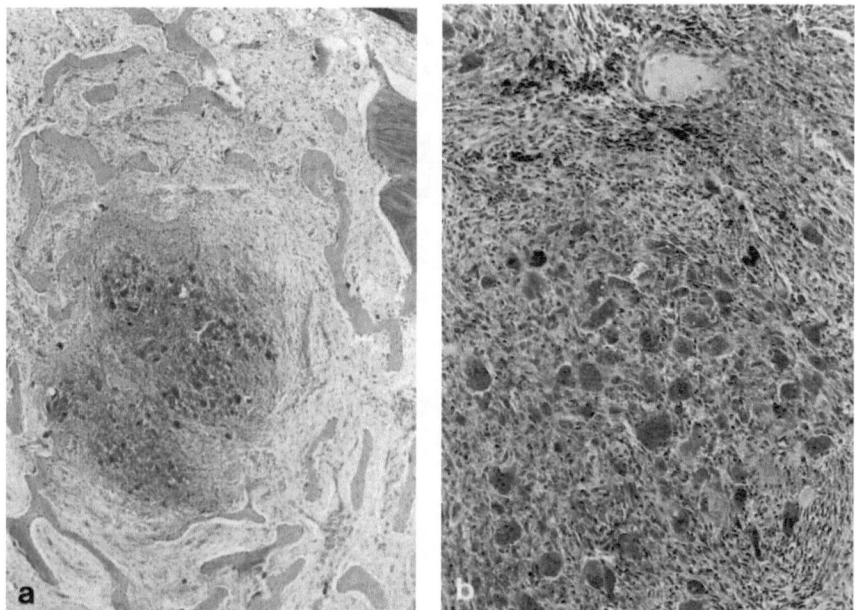

Fig. 164 a, b. *Brown tumour of hyperparathyroidism.* Same case as Fig. 163

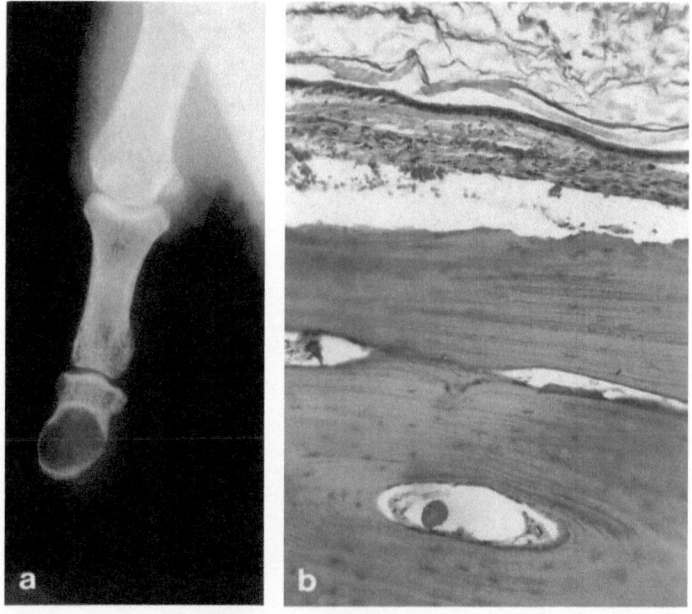

Fig. 165 a, b. *Intraosseous epidermoid cyst.* **a** Female, 38 years. Distal phalanx of finger. Radiograph. **b** Intraosseous epidermoid cyst

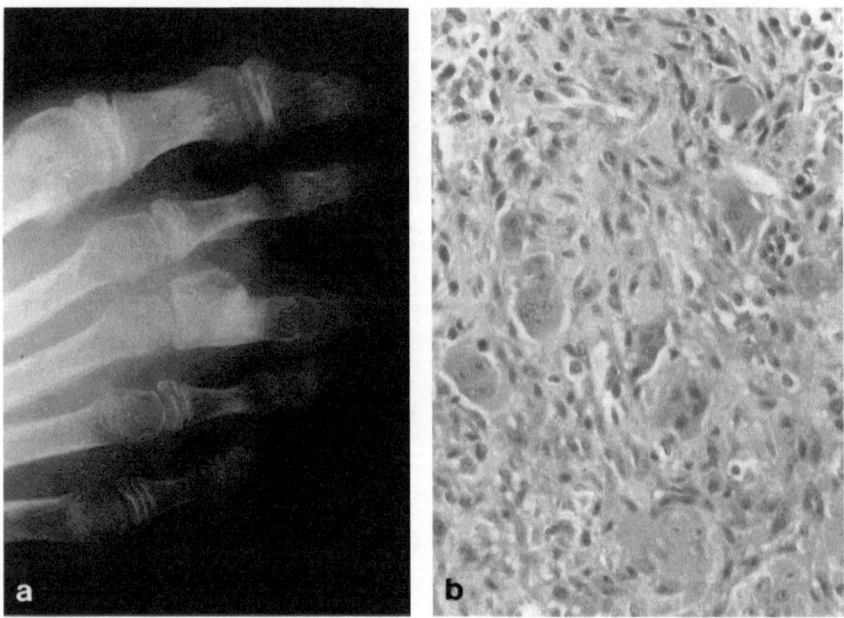

Fig. 166 a, b. *Giant-cell (reparative) granuloma.* **a** Female, 12 years. Proximal phalanx, third toe. Radiograph. **b** Giant-cell (reparative) granuloma

Subject Index

 **World Health Organization**
International Histological Classification of Tumours

P. Kleihues, P. C. Burger,
B. W. Scheithauer

Histological Typing of Tumours of the Central Nervous System

Co-Author: L. H. Sobin
2nd ed. 1993. XIV, 112 pp. 106 figs. in color. (WHO-International Histological Classification of Tumours.
Ed.: L. H. Sobin)
ISBN 3-540-56971-5

I. R. H. Kramer, J. J. Pindborg,
M. Shear

Histological Typing of Odontogenic Tumours

2nd ed. 1992. XI, 118 pp. 142 figs.
(WHO-International Histological Classification of Tumours. Ed.: L. H. Sobin)
ISBN 3-540-54142-X

C. Hedinger
Histological Typing of Thyroid Tumours

In Collaboration with E. D. Williams
and L. H. Sobin
2nd ed. 1988. XII, 67 pp. 92 figs.
ISBN 3-540-19244-1

H. Watanabe, J. R. Jass, L. H. Sobin

Histological Typing of Oesophageal and Gastric Tumours

2nd ed. 1990. XII, 109 pp. 120 figs.
4 tabs. ISBN 3-540-51629-8

K. Shanmugaratnam

Histological Typing of Tumours of the Upper Respiratory Tract and Ear

In Collaboration with L. H. Sobin
2nd ed. 1991. XI, 201 pp. 200 figs.
ISBN 3-540-53880-1

G. Seifert

Histological Typing of Salivary Gland Tumours

In Collaboration with L. H. Sobin
2nd ed. 1991. XI, 113 pp. 124 figs.
2 tabs. ISBN 3-540-54031-8

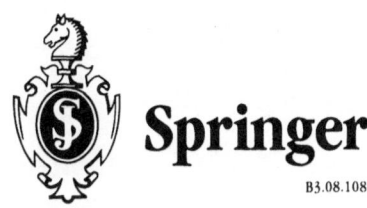 Springer

B3.08.108